Finally, a diet that's JUST FOR ME!

Finally, a diet that's JUST FOR ME!

YOUR GUIDE TO A HEALTHIER LIFE

Introducing

The JustForMeDiet

Janessa Grady Fleming

Foreword by Joseph R. Robinson, M.D., Ph.D

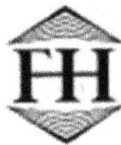

Foundation House Publishing, LLC

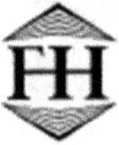

Foundation House Publishing, LLC
Contact: www.foundationhousepublishing.com
Email at: thejustformediet@gmail.com

ISBN: 0986423904
ISBN 13: 9780986423901
Library of Congress Control Number: 2015900273
Foundation House Publishing, Silver Spring, MD
Illustrations by Daniel Stephens
Author photography by John Nelson, Artist

Acknowledgements

I first thank GOD for His goodness, guidance, and the grace needed to write this book. To Mitchell, my loving and supportive husband – your steadfastness, suggestions, and sanity have allowed me to see this project to completion. To my brilliant son, Vincent – your encouragement and enthusiasm kept me edified throughout this journey. I also thank my parents, Paul and Carrie Grady, who always champion and cheerlead their children and grandchildren – thank you for being a wealth of wisdom and a deep well of unwavering love. To my parents-in-law, Edward and Elsie Fleming – thank you for constant care and concern for me and my family.

Many thanks to my insightful and irreplaceable brothers, Kevin, Paul, Jr., and Jendayo Grady, Ph.D, and many thanks to my brothers and sisters-in-law for your unfeigned love and loyalty. To Joseph R. Robinson, M.D., Ph.D., thank you for your medical care and for motivating me to move more often, to mind my "peas and carrots," and to memorialize this weight loss and healthy living journey. To Reverend Lionel P. Pointer, Pastor of the Round Oak Missionary Baptist Church and first lady Dr. Michelle Pointer – thank you for your spiritual sustenance, strength and stability.

Finally, to all those who shared their experiences with me, stepped out on faith to try the *JustForMeDiet*, suggested topics for inclusion, and supported this project – a million thanks!

Dedication

This book is for the working mother, the church deacon, the former athlete, the desk jockey, the sedentary, the overworked retiree, the single mom, the long commuter, the "sick and tired of being sick and tired," the "tired of cookie-cutter diets," and everyone else who has no time, no money, no energy, no trainer, and no hope of losing weight and reclaiming good health. The *JustForMeDiet* is for *you!*

Table of Contents

Disclaimer

The contents of this book, including text, graphics, images, and other material, are for informational purposes only. This book does not contain medical advice and is not intended to be a substitute for informed professional medical or mental advice, care, diagnosis, or treatment of any health problems or illnesses. Any questions regarding your own physical or mental health or the health of your children should be addressed to your own physician or other health care provider. You should not use this information to diagnose or treat any health problems or illnesses without consulting your pediatrician or family doctor. Please consult a doctor with any questions or concerns you might have regarding your or your children's health or medical condition. Nothing in this book is intended to cause you to delay consulting with or seeking treatment from your physician or medical care provider or visiting an emergency room in the event of a medical emergency. Consult your physician or medical care provider before applying or adopting any suggestion found in this book. Do not begin any treatment, medication, or supplement as a result of something you read in this book, and do not cease any treatment, medication, or supplement as a result of something you read in this book without first consulting your physician or health care provider. The author and publisher of this book make no warranties or representations regarding the accuracy or usefulness to anyone other than the author of the information contained herein. The author and publisher of this book assume no risk or liability in connection with the use of the information contained herein. While the nutritional information for the product brands referenced herein was accurate as of the date of this book's publication, product manufacturers routinely change their ingredients and nutritional labels. Therefore, do not rely on the nutritional information contained herein as your only source of product information, but consult the websites or nutritional labels of the products themselves for the most up to date and accurate sources of the product's nutritional information.

Foreword

t is my distinct pleasure and honor to be invited by the author, Janessa Grady Fleming, to write the foreword on what I believe will be a wonderful and meaningful addition to the reader's library of very stimulating and educational discourses. As the title, *Finally, A Diet That's Just For Me* suggests, this is the chronicle of the author's journey to weight loss and a healthy lifestyle. In some small way throughout her writing, she refers to her "Doctor" as a motivating influence. Before continuing, allow me to reminisce a bit.

I have had the pleasure of being the physician for the entire family for greater than forty years. This includes her parents, siblings, and most recently, her son. During this time, I have seen her evolve into a very skilled and highly motivated individual. I could not be more proud of her and her accomplishments, which include being an attorney, minister, and now an author who unfolds in this book her personal quest to achieving excellent health.

It was during one of her visits to me that we discussed the current state of African-American health, and the impact of obesity, in particular, on the state of African-American health. We also discussed the lack of emphasis on controlling this most devastating disease – yes, disease, a most preventable disease in this country. At that time, I related to her a video, recently released by the Association of Black Cardiologists, that chronicled the role of the black church and "what we eat" in the fight to overcome obesity. Perhaps it was during that visit that I may have "inadvertently" suggested that her BMI (Body Mass Index) was a bit out of the range of "healthy."

As you follow the author's weight loss journey that, ultimately, lays the foundation for the *JustForMeDiet*, a few facts about obesity are to be appreciated:

- As of 2014, nearly thirty-five percent of U.S. adults and seventeen percent of children and adolescents have obesity.
- As of the fall of 2014, the American Heart Association (AHA), the American College of Cardiology (ACC), The Obesity Society (TOS), and the World Health Organization (WHO) all emphasized that obesity causes more deaths than smoking, and is now the leading cause of preventable deaths in the world.

As a physician, one of my roles is to counsel patients toward incorporating physical activity and healthier eating habits into their lives. This counseling is critical to successful intervention to control the number one cause of preventable deaths. I often tell my patients, "You are what you eat!" Heart disease, stroke, type 2 diabetes, and certain cancers all could be reduced with appropriate weight loss and exercising. It is heartwarming when your patients successfully apply the wellness guidance you have provided to improve their lives.

Lifestyle modification, physical activity, and most importantly, outstanding and motivational stories will be revealed throughout *Finally, A Diet That's Just For Me*. This book should contribute mightily to a successful journey to better health and a better quality of life. For this, I applaud her and highly recommend this treatise for your reading pleasure. It will be a fun and a magnificent voyage to better health and both quality and quantity of life.

Joseph R. Robinson, MD, Ph.D., FAP, FACC

Introduction

**Beloved, I pray that you may prosper in all things
and be in health, just as your soul prospers.**
3 JOHN 2 (NKJV)

f you are like me, you have been on the losing end of the weight-loss battle for years. For women, weight loss was about keeping our girlish figures; for guys, maintaining the six-pack abs from their youth was important. Now the doctor has told you to lose the weight or risk losing your life. The warning that "you have to lose fifty pounds or else" is frightening, of course, but it is meaningless when you have tried every diet plan out there with no lasting success. The doctor's words only add to the stress.

Nonetheless, the doctor warns you that your weight problem is the reason you now have prediabetes or full-onset diabetes and are at risk for cancer and cardiovascular disease. The weight is the reason you had knee surgery, why your feet swell all the time, why your cousin retired on disability, and why your back hurts all the time. It's why you can't catch a breath walking up the stairs, and why it hurts to walk down those same stairs. The weight is why you have high blood pressure and must now take medicine that makes you dizzy and bloated all the time. And if the doctor's warning isn't bad enough, the worst part of all is that you wonder if things will ever change. No one else seems to be able to shed the weight—maybe this is how it's supposed to be. You and everyone else you know have paid big bucks for those unbreakable gym membership contracts. You have tried Pilates and kick-boxing, taken Garcinia this and ketones that. You've been drinking umpteen bottles of water a day and replaced meat with soy—all to no avail.

Success Starts Today!

Starting today, your past weight-loss failures are a thing of the past. Yes, your prayers have been answered. After all, "With GOD all things are possible." You *can* drop your weight, high blood pressure, elevated blood sugar, cancer risk, and high cholesterol. You can regain your energy, youthfulness, confidence, and health. This book is going to take you by the hand and lead you along the path to weight-loss success. By following the *JustForMeDiet*, you will lose the weight—tons of it! I lost forty-five pounds, and so can you.

You will learn how to discard unhealthy eating and living habits and how to pave a personalized path to a slimmer you. After all, your body is one of a kind. Your health needs individualized care, and you have the keys to the kingdom. Your health requires an inward look and focus. It is about you. Tell yourself, this journey is going to be about me...*just for me*!

This diet is all about you!

This diet is called the *JustForMeDiet* because it is time to deal with you. You've taken care of everyone else around you and have been quite successful at saving the world. You have invested all of your time and energy into everyone but you and have left no time to care for yourself. After all, that's what we've been taught to do. However, what good are you to your family, friends, church, or job—or yourself—if you are always sick, tired, or worn out? Well, this book shows you how to lose weight and regain your energy and vitality, and it lays the foundation for lasting health. Only then can you be at your best for those around you. To love those around you, you need to be alive and well. So...Welcome to the *JustForMeDiet*!

Why other diets might fail

Indeed, for far too long, we have followed this diet or that fad with no lasting success. We spend tens of billions of dollars in diet and weight-loss supplements and programs each year. There are hundreds of diet programs and plans, pills, supplements, sprinkles, drinks, wraps, gyms, products, and meals. Sadly, we are more overweight and obese than ever before. Why is that? It is because we have not zeroed in on the reasons why we are gaining weight in the first place. This book exposes some of the eye-opening factors that collide to create the perfect storm of weight gain and disease in this country. Prime examples include the hefty contribution our sedentary state adds to our weight problem, hormones and antibiotics fed to our livestock, and even the plastic water bottles we drink from on a daily basis. Second, we want tailor-fitted success with an off-the-rack product. That wedding dress or tuxedo is fitted, refitted, and altered to perfection because your body is so uniquely curved and shaped such that professional tailoring is your only hope of obtaining the perfect fit. I am sure that most of us can agree that:

- Many diets are one size fits all and cannot factor your medically based food restrictions.
- Some diet pills have been linked to liver damage and/or an increased risk of a cardiovascular disease (CVD) event, such as a heart attack or stroke.
- Many diet plans make unrealistic promises unconcerned with your nutritional needs: "Just take this pill or sprinkle this magic powder and

you can eat all the pizza and cake you want and still lose weight!" You just might lose the weight, but you could develop diabetes, raise your blood pressure, and increase your risk of CVD. Are you willing to take that risk? Also, are you going to take diet pills for the rest of your life? Are you going to be a lifelong "sprinkler"? Of course not.

- Some diet plans want you to buy prepackaged foods that the rest of your family will not eat (or can't afford to eat).

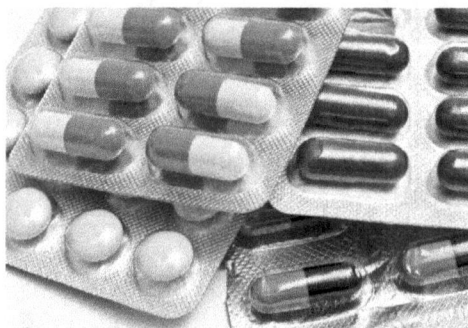

By showing you how to develop your own *JustForMeDiet*—a diet that is tailored to you, your medical history, food allergies, age, budget limitations, schedule, and even taste buds—you *can* lose the weight and regain your life. Indeed, this transformative book cracks the code to the food puzzle and identifies many of the surprise hindrances and weight-loss saboteurs that keep you from losing weight. You will learn how to spot and eliminate those saboteurs. Finally, this book will offer dozens of suggestions, alternatives, nutritional guidelines, meal plan ideas, and damage-control techniques that should help your body shed the weight and keep it off!

MY STORY

Before I unknowingly began developing the *JustForMeDiet*, my doctor cautioned me about my weight. He explained that my Body Mass Index, or BMI, was in the obese range. What? No one ever told me I was obese. He also told me I needed to lose *at least* thirty pounds. That's not so terrible when you are eighteen years old. Try losing thirty pounds when you are around fifty years old (oops! Did I just say that?), have a long commute, have a family, love to eat all the wrong foods, are addicted to bread and French fries, and have a sweet tooth. You *know* thirty pounds isn't easy. But I did it! I even lost fifteen more pounds. So can you. Interestingly, along the way I noticed people would tell me: "Oh, you look great!" Or, "You don't need to lose any more weight. You don't want to become anorexic!" As if that could ever happen to someone who eats as much as I do. I had a better chance of winning the lottery than losing "too much" weight. I realized, however, that most people judge weight-loss needs by the person's appearance. The problem with that assessment tool is that we have adopted a new normal for what is a healthy weight. We now are used to seeing much larger-sized Americans than in decades past; what used to be overweight now appears normal or on the small side. That's why the BMI scale is so important—it keeps it real. (See Body Mass Index Table in Appendix A)

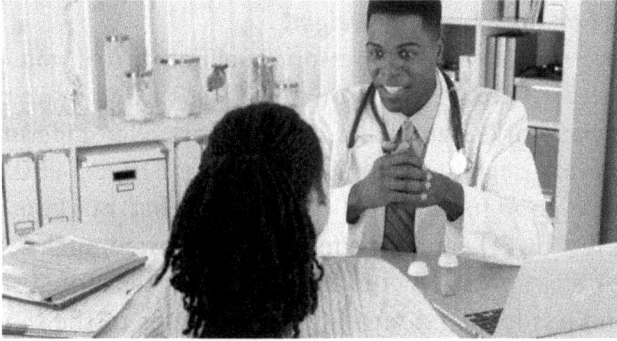

Increased Weight = Increased Risk of Diabetes

Back to the doctor's news: As if hearing "obese" wasn't bad enough, I learned that my A1C was slightly elevated. Huh? My A1 *what* was elevated? Isn't that a steak sauce? He explained that the A1C measures the amount of glucose in my hemoglobin and is a predictor of diabetes. Yes, the dreaded D word. I was approaching the pre-D-word level. This news sounded the alarm for a couple of reasons: first, an increased risk of cardiovascular disease accompanies pre-D; and second, a few years ago, I had a friend who suffered from diabetes. She had a stroke and became partially blind. One day she called to say she'd be cooking her last Easter dinner because she would not live to see another Easter. She warned that if my doctor ever tells me to lose weight or risk contracting diabetes, I should lose the weight. She went on to say that, "I didn't listen to my doctor. I figured that, hey, this is the food Momma and Grandma were both raised on, and they turned out okay, so that doctor doesn't know what he's talking about. I'm just 'big-boned.' Well, I was wrong, and I know this will be my last Easter dinner." It *was* her last Easter.

Lose the weight and lose the pain.

I promised her I would listen to my doctor. I encourage all of you to do the same. I now am forty-five, yes, *forty-five pounds lighter*: from 186 to 141 pounds, at five feet six and a half. (Excuse me, but I need to do the happy dance!) I have much more energy, my thoughts are clearer, my knees do not hurt anymore, and neither does my back. No more bloating. No more sleeping after meals. No more being too tired to do anything after work except to collapse! Now, I want to share my journey to this healthier and lighter existence along with the secret to creating your own *JustForMeDiet* plan. You, too, can be the slimmer, healthier person GOD created you to be.

I am an expert on how I lost my weight!

So what makes me, an average person, qualified to tell you how to lose weight? That's easy. I am an expert on how *I* lost the forty-five pounds. Like you, I know what worked and what did not work over a lifetime. Like you, I have an honorary degree in eating and dieting. I have a PhD in "carbing" out. I know what good food tastes like. Not only that, but I put my doctor's advice to the test by (1) eating the foods he suggested, such as oatmeal for breakfast as often as possible, nuts and peanut butter, more fish, fruits, and vegetables, and less fatty red meat; (2) saying adios to the foods he called inflammatory, including refined foods, fast food, fried foods, sugar, white rice, and potatoes, and most bread products; and (3) buying a pedometer to ensure I'm taking a minimum of ten thousand steps per day. I also accessed and gathered valuable information and guidance from the Centers for Disease Control and Prevention (CDC), Health.gov, and other valuable resources. I applied that information to my eating and unhealthy lifestyle habits, ultimately, to create a customizable and effective weight loss plan that was just for me. I shared the plan with family and friends and, lo and behold, they made the plan their own and lost weight, too. With a range of twenty to forty pounds lost thus far per person, my family and friends are becoming slimmer and trimmer by the minute. It worked for me, it worked for others, and it can work for you!

How do I make this diet just for me?

I'm glad you asked. Because *you* are an expert on your body, you know your food allergies, medications, medical history, schedule, disabilities, etc. *You*, and not a one-size-fits-all diet, need to be the one to choose the foods, snacks, and beverages you are allowed to eat and drink. The *JustForMeDiet* allows you to choose food items from a very carefully compiled list of foods and beverages that work synergistically to maximize your weight loss.

Whether for breakfast, lunch, dinner, or snacks, you need certain food combinations to maximize the weight loss—permanently! Not everyone can eat all the foods in each of these groups. Therefore, this diet provides a variety of food items from which to choose to build your meals. You pick the foods you're *not* allergic to; you choose the foods that do *not* interfere with your medicines. One item from each meal list should meet your requirements and restrictions. Simultaneously, for those who want a ready-made meal plan, this book provides "A Week in the Life" of the *JustForMeDiet* as an example of how to build meal plans that contain a healthy combination of the macronutrients needed for healthy weight loss. Feel free to use it. Feel free to create your own "Week in the Life" meal plan. Finally, as you begin to apply the *JustForMeDiet* to your life, you will discover that this book really leads to a lifestyle change. This change necessarily includes declaring war on being sedentary. But there's no condemnation here. We're all in this together.

I lost the weight without the gym!

Experts agree that we need to engage in four to five thirty-minute sets of exercise per week. If you have the time, resources, and commitment to accomplish your exercise routine in a structured setting, such as the gym or the recreation center's Zumba class, by all means do so. This exercise requirement, however, can be met simply by walking regularly throughout the day, doing "deskercises," performing regular household chores, playing with the kids, or even gardening. The key is to engage in physical activity or movement throughout the day. You don't need to pay a gym through the nose for the next ten years to accomplish these regular movement sets. You need only to stand up and move! Of course, the thirty minute set remains the gold standard, but you will discover there are a variety of ways to implement that recommendation.

This book will provide several effective alternatives to traditional, often cost-prohibitive exercise plans that may be inconvenient, too difficult at your age, overwhelming, burdensome, or simply not practical.

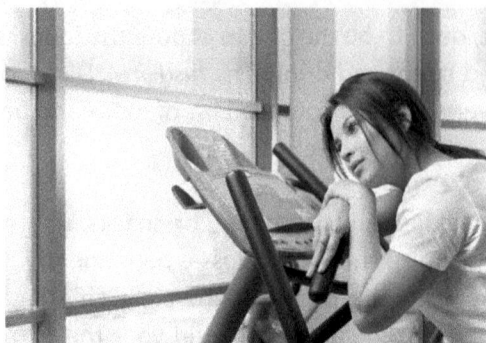

The JustForMe Tips

As you turn the pages of this book, you will discover tips, substitutes, and alternatives you can apply to your particular dietary restrictions and physical limitations. Examples include:

- I have trouble sleeping at night (chapter 2).
- I can't walk thirty minutes all at once (chapter 2).
- I have no way to heat up leftovers at work (chapter 2).
- My kids won't eat healthy cereal (chapter 4).
- I am allergic to nuts (chapter 5).
- Stevia upsets my stomach (chapter 5).
- I am allergic to dairy products (chapter 6).
- I am on blood thinners and cannot eat greens (chapter 6).
- Someone else does my grocery shopping (chapter 6).
- I don't have a refrigerator at work (chapter 6).
- I have fibroid tumors (chapter 6).
- I have acid reflux and can't drink water with lemons (chapter 7).
- I have really bad knees (chapter 10).
- My job (receptionist, psychologist) requires me to sit all day (chapter 10).
- I can't afford to buy organic food (chapter 11).
- How do I know which foods contain GMOs? (chapter 11).
- I cannot fast because I'm on medication (chapter 12).

So let us begin this transformative journey designed to change your health and life for the better!

CHAPTER 1

Common Weight-Loss Myths

And the truth shall set you free.
JOHN 8:32

Before we get started, we need to explore some of the myths perpetuating our inability to lose the weight and keep it off.

MYTH #1: *The BMI scale doesn't apply to me.*
How many times have we used that excuse? According to the CDC, calculating Body Mass Index (BMI)[i] is one of the best methods for population assessment of overweight and obesity. So I'm sorry, but the BMI scale does apply to us. BMI is a measure of body fat for men and women, based on height and weight. The scale provides a high/low range of acceptable BMIs with the corresponding weights. It allows for both thin- and heavy-boned bodies. For example, the normal BMI range for a woman who measures five feet six inches tall is 18.5–24.9. The corresponding weight for that range is 118–155 pounds, nearly a forty-pound differential. We need to take that range seriously because it just might save our lives. For your reference, please consult the Body Mass Index Table in Appendix A.

MYTH #2: *As long as I count my calories, it doesn't matter what I eat.*
In fact, it really does matter how you get those calories. Yes, dropping calories (but not too many) is a proven weight-loss strategy. However, consuming too many carbohydrates and sugars interferes with the proper metabolism of the fat you are trying to shed, regardless of how many calories you give up. During my weight-loss success, I did not count calories. Instead, I counted carbohydrates, sugars, fiber, fat, and protein. Nevertheless, for you calorie counters out there,

my doctor told me that a good guide for calorie counting is simply to add a zero to your weight and not to exceed that many calories. For example, if you weigh two hundred pounds, to lose weight you must not exceed two thousand calories per day. Conventional wisdom says that to lose weight, you need to subtract four to five hundred calories per day. Again, my weight-loss success was *not* calorie driven. It happened when I stopped eating processed food, sugars, fried food, junk food, and trans fats, and when I began to eat fiber, protein, and good fat.

MYTH #3: *People can't lose weight because they are lazy, have no willpower, and eat too much!*

Actually, there are many reasons why millions of us can't lose weight. These include being sedentary, genetics, depression, medications, disabilities, food addictions, and toxic overload. As you can see, some of these factors are beyond a person's control. This book will help you accept the things you can't change (genes), and it will show you how to navigate around the factors beyond your control to focus on what you can change. I want to make it clear that I did not lose forty-five pounds based on willpower. No, I lost those pounds by keeping the food temptation from plain view and by following the steps that have been described for you in these pages.

MYTH #4: *You have to eliminate all fat from your diet to lose weight.*

The truth is, we need fat in our diet—even if you want to lose weight. My grand-mother used to tell me that I need *some* fat. Well, Grandma was right, as usual! There are bad fats and there are good fats. Later on, I'll show you why good fats are a key piece of the weight-loss puzzle.

MYTH #5: *Drinking juices instead of sodas is a sure way to begin to lose the weight.*

OMG! In my opinion, juices and juice drinks are worse than drinking soda because they give us a false sense of security. First, everyone knows that sodas are loaded with sugar and phosphoric acid. I knew soda was bad when someone poured cola—no need to name which brand—on my car battery to get rid of corrosion. Second, most fruit juices have as much, if not more, sugars and calories than soda. The sugar enters the bloodstream directly, causing sugar spikes and weight gain. Let them go. It is always better to eat the whole fruit if you can.

MYTH #6: *A diet's success is measured by how quickly the weight is shed.*

Although an initial weight loss of about ten to fifteen pounds during the first two to three weeks can be a good way to jump-start your weight-loss adventure, trying to sustain that speed of weight loss for the long haul actually can be dangerous.

My doctor informed me it was medically necessary for me to lose at least thirty pounds. On the *JustForMeDiet* I lost thirty pounds in the first 120 days. After that, I no longer had a sense of urgency because I had reached the "medical necessity weight." I took my time to lose the last fifteen pounds to reach my goal of 141 pounds - down from 186! I took my time for another reason. I wanted to keep it off. Despite my own pace, I don't want to promise that "You'll lose fifty pounds in fifty minutes!" Let's face it, who doesn't want to lose fifty pounds in fifty minutes—sounds catchy, doesn't it? Like a nice book title: *Lose Fifty Pounds in Fifty Minutes!* I'm sure there's one out there. Losing weight too quickly often requires dietary deprivation and exercise overload. It may be dangerous to maintain over the long haul, and the weight usually returns as quickly as it was lost. Then there's the saggy skin. Need I say more? So please don't try to lose fifty pounds in fifty minutes, or in fifty days for that matter. If you lose fifty pounds in six to nine months, you have cause to celebrate! I lost the thirty that my physician told me to lose to reach the top of my BMI range in four months. That was fast enough. Besides, *the race is not to the swift...*

The point is that you will lose the weight at a pace that is good for your body. Your body is not the enemy, and it will work with you if you treat it right.

MYTH #7: *I must eliminate all carbohydrates from my diet to lose weight.*
Nothing could be further from the truth. Yes, we need carbohydrates (let's call them "carbs"), but in addition to lowering the number of carbs, we need to change the *types* of carbs we eat. According to www.womenshealth.gov,[ii] there are three types of carbs—sugars, starches, and dietary fibers. Sugars and starches convert to glucose, or blood sugar, which actually provides energy for red blood cells and the brain. Although we're supposed to burn off excess glucose, middle-aged sedentary Americans no longer burn off these excess sugars. The results? Obesity, diabetes, cardiovascular disease, diabetes, and an increased risk of cancer.

Contrast those sugars and empty starches to the "fiber carbs." These are some of the *good* carbs. They rid the intestines of excess fats (I can stop right there!), slow digestion and help reduce sugar spikes. Everyone knows that fiber also makes us feel full, so we don't overeat. Foods high in fiber include fruits (including avocados), vegetables, beans, peas, nuts, seeds, whole-grain foods, oatmeal, and brown rice. I ate these healthy carbs with every meal and snack throughout my weight-loss odyssey.

MYTH #8: *It doesn't matter what I eat as long as I burn it off when I go to the gym.*

I used to believe that myth until I failed to lose weight even after training for a triathlon. For eight weeks I swam, biked, and jogged *every day*—and lost virtually no weight by the end of the race (start weight: 182; end weight: 180) because I had been overloading on fiber-less, nutrient-deficient carbohydrates that caused sugar spikes and insulin resistance. Also, I was sedentary throughout the day except for the one "workout" hour. I have since learned that the one hour of working out does not offset the negative health consequences of sitting for the rest of the day. Once I learned to move throughout the day and to change what I ate, the weight poured off. Yours will, too!

CHAPTER 2

Slim and Trim Start Today!

Weeping may endure for a night, but joy comes in the morning.
PSALM 30:5

Congratulations! No matter what you currently weigh, and regardless of your current size or shape, the metamorphosis to the slimmer, trimmer, and healthier you is already underway. You will succeed! So let's get down to business.

. . .

If your goal is to lose thirty, forty, or even fifty pounds, and keep it off, you first must decide to make you and your health *the* priorities for the foreseeable future. Just as having a baby results in a wonderful but significant change to your life, so is the advanced preparation required to lose the weight, keep it off, and regain some health along the way. Your weight-loss success depends on your willingness to let go of negative eating habits, and to develop new ways of studying nutrition labels and ingredient lists. Since what we eat and drink is directly linked to weight gain or weight loss, we need to know precisely what we are eating and drinking. Make sense? Your success involves letting go of certain foods, but it also involves trying new and more wholesome foods, perhaps for the first time. Far too often I hear, "Oh, I don't like [this or that food]." Seriously, that phrase should be phased out of your speech for the time being. Now, before we jump into the *JustForMeDiet* plan, we need to take a few minutes to explore why we failed at losing weight in the past. Most of the reasons why I couldn't lose weight are on this list.

Why haven't I lost the weight?

If you are like me, for years you dieted, ate rabbit food, worked out in the gym , tried triathlons, skipped meals, drank diet sodas and experimented with various diet programs, with little to no success. Or, you lost some weight and then gained it all back with a few more pounds to spare (more like a spare tire!). You never really understood why you experienced so little success. This chapter explores some of the hindrances to your weight-loss success and overall health. No matter what you do, as long as these problems are in your way, your weight loss will be minimal. By the way, no single factor was responsible for my weight gain over the years. The heavy carbs alone did not do it. Sitting all day, by itself, was not why I picked up dozens of pounds. Toxic overload, alone, was not the culprit either. It was the combination of these factors, including genetics, stressors, and bad choices over a lifetime that created that perfect storm of weight gain and increased my risk of serious chronic diseases. Below I single out some of those culprits. So, let's explore ten very real reasons many of us have trouble losing the weight:

The top ten reasons why I couldn't lose the weight

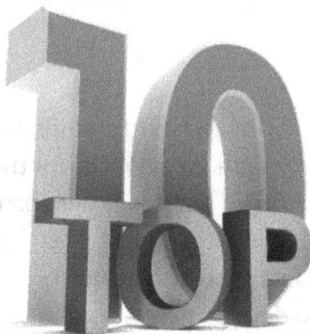

1. **SITTING ALL DAY**: Also called the "sitting disease," whether you are sitting for hours at the computer, at meetings, at your kids' games, in front of the TV, or on planes, trains, and in automobiles, trouble is just around the corner. Recently, health experts began equating sitting all day to the dangerous effects of smoking. The alarming connection between extended periods of uninterrupted sitting and diabetes, cancer, and cardiovascular disease will be explained later on in chapter 10. If you change nothing else, stand up and walk around your house, apartment or office even as you read this book. I learned to incorporate the "two-minute drill" into my daily life—every thirty minutes, I try to stand up

and move for two minutes. You'll see the drill from time to time in this book—when you see it, stand and walk for at least two minutes...or longer!

2. **EATING PROCESSED/REFINED FOODS**: We eat way too many processed and overly-carbed food "products": nutrient-deprived bread, crackers, potato chips, pizza (I know, blasphemy!), breakfast cereals - even the self-proclaimed healthy ones, cookies, cakes, pies and other desserts, many muffins, doughnuts, and other foods with a high-glycemic load. The glycemic load measures a food's impact on a person's rise in blood sugar—the higher the load, the worse for you and me.

3. **CONSUMING OBESOGENS IN OUR FOOD, WATER BOTTLES, CANS, AND PERSONAL-CARE PRODUCTS**: Yes, "obesogens" is a term that refers to the chemicals in our foods and personal-care products, among other things, thought by many researchers to cause our bodies to make and store fat cells.

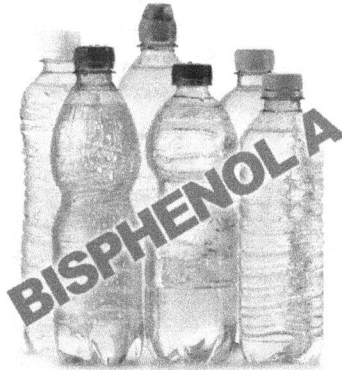

Examples of potential obesogens include, but are not limited to: (1) Bisphenol A, or BPA, a chemical used in many of our plastic water bottles and canned food linings; (2) antibiotics and growth hormones given to the livestock that provide our meat and dairy products; (3) pesticides used on our produce; (4) pesticides that are genetically engineered into the DNA of our foods; and (5) phthalates, parabens, sodium lauryl sulfates, and other chemicals used in many toothpastes, hair and body products, and perfumes and colognes.

4. **DRINKING LIQUID SUGAR**: We can drink our way fat or we can drink our way slim. Sodas, fancy coffee drinks, fruit juices (yes, our beloved OJ), sweet teas, store-bought smoothie drinks, and many cocktails are all loaded in

sugar, carbs, and calories. There are more calories, carbohydrates, and sugars in some twenty-ounce bottles of soda than there are in a serving of apple pie and ice cream. Lose the liquid sugar and the pounds will pour off!

5. **EATING TOO MUCH UNHEALTHY FAT, AND NOT ENOUGH FIBER AND PROTEIN:** The dietary pitfall here involved subsisting on a diet that was void of fiber, healthy fat, and protein. On the other hand, successful weight loss involves developing a diet that is filled with those macronutrients, otherwise known as the "healthy trinity." These macronutrients work to minimize sugar spikes, assist the body with metabolizing nutrients, provide energy and fat burning, and help to control insulin. Consuming the required daily amounts of these macronutrients is a must if you want to lose weight.

6. **EATING OUTSIDE OF THE HOME:** For some of us, this can constitute 40–50 percent or more of our meals. Many of us actually shop for and prepare healthy meals to eat at home but end up eating out more often than not. This is the battlefield where the war on our weight potentially is won or lost.

7. **ENDURING PRESSURE FROM FAMILY AND FRIENDS/NO WEIGHT LOSS SUPPORT NETWORK:** Family buy-in is essential to your success; otherwise, your efforts will be hindered. I have discovered that the one way to minimize this pressure is to help those closest to me to adopt healthier eating habits and lifestyles. You might feel pressured by family and friends to eat the unhealthy foods they prepare, or to eat unhealthy restaurant foods. For weight-loss success, however, you must avoid eating foods that don't support a healthy weight.

8. **BEING SLEEP DEPRIVED:** There is a direct link between our poor sleeping habits and weight gain.[iii] The less you sleep, the less weight you lose. Our physicians tell us that most adults need somewhere between seven to eight hours of sleep per night. This is proving more difficult these days because the LED lights on our televisions, computers, and cell phones disrupt our natural sleep patterns. Our body's ability to make melatonin—the chemical that helps us to sleep—decreases.[iv] When that happens, we gain weight.

9. **NOT PRIORITIZING HEALTH:** When I ate on the run, ate out regularly, or bought prepared or processed food products that promised quick and easy meals, I was missing the boat and was destined to be fat. Yes, I said fat. I realized that to lose the weight and regain my health, I needed to reorder my priorities and carve out time for my health and for the health of my family. This involved setting aside time to plan meals and snacks, studying nutrition labels, reading ingredients, comparing prices, and fitting walks and other "movement" breaks into my schedule.

10. **BEING UNWILLING TO CHANGE:** When I share with friends and family the weight-loss generating foods I incorporated into my diet, often the response is a surprising, "Well, I don't like oatmeal" or "I don't like guacamole" or "I can't live without my..." (you finish the sentence). Believe me, I understand. This process involves transition which doesn't happen overnight. Keep in mind, however, that food's purpose isn't solely to satisfy or stimulate our taste buds. Food should provide nourishment and healing to the body and mind, not the diseases caused by so many of the foods we have been eating. We must ensure that our foods are serving their holistic purpose. Let's aim to strike that healthy balance going forward.

I know what you're thinking...Wow! That list is heavy duty. Where do I even begin? Relax. As you turn the pages of this book, the yellow brick road map will come into view, and you will learn proven techniques to navigate a smooth transition from the weight-loss and health hindrances to the weight-loss success you need for maximum health.

****

JUSTFORME TIP: I Have Trouble Sleeping at Night
Powering down an hour before bed, which includes turning off the television, computer, and cell phone, will make a huge difference. I drink chamomile tea or one ounce of tart cherry juice at bedtime because it is loaded with melatonin. When I do so, I'm out like a light within fifteen minutes!
****

The Ten Commandments for losing the first ten pounds

Now that we have explored the top-ten reasons why many of us can't lose the weight, here are my top-ten strategies that melted off the first ten pounds in less than three weeks! Before I began the *JustForMeDiet*, it would take me two months to lose four pounds, only to gain it back in two weeks. I followed the *JustForMeDiet* guidelines faithfully and without exception, and the results were thrilling! Faithful adherence to this plan was necessary to jump-start the weight loss and sugar purge. My body needed a shocking change to jolt it into fat-burning mode. Although that shock did not include running sprints or eliminating all carbohydrates, it did involve purchasing a pedometer the day before Thanksgiving. I hoped to achieve my goal of ten thousand steps beginning that day, and every day thereafter (including Thanksgiving Day)—no exceptions. The first ten pounds poured off when I followed these actions:

(1) Taking a minimum of ten thousand steps per day, which included standing up every twenty to thirty minutes to walk or move for at least two minutes;

(2) Eliminating fast-food breakfasts, lunches, or dinners *entirely*;

(3) Cutting out most breads, rolls, biscuits, pancakes, waffles, bagels, sweets, cold cereal, granola bars, most crackers, pizza, white potatoes, white rice, and most pasta *with few exceptions*;

(4) Restricting my carbohydrate intake to around one hundred grams per day for a few weeks while correcting my protein, fiber and healthy fat imbalance;

(5) Eliminating beverages with sugar (natural or added) and chemical artificial sweeteners *completely*, including juices or juice drinks, sodas, and diet sodas;

(6) Switching to one teaspoon of coconut sugar or organic stevia as my added sweetener;

(7) Eating three to five servings of fruits and vegetables every day;

(8) Drinking seven to eight glasses of water and/or herbal tea every day;

(9) Using vinaigrette dressing exclusively on my salads, which I ate three to four times per week; and

(10) Not cheating, no matter what tempting foods my well-meaning family and friends offered.

A FEW MORE STARTING THOUGHTS...

Pray for help!

We already know that GOD wants us to be whole and healthy, and He promised that if we ask, we will receive. After a lifetime of failure in my own strength in regard to weight loss, I realized I needed divine intervention (seriously!). So I asked GOD for help. I started with, *Lord, please help me to lose this weight!* Along the way, I added situational prayers such as, *Lord, please help me exercise self-control at the birthday dinner or other food-filled event.* I expanded my prayer further with, *Lord, please help me to resist temptation,* and *pick me up when (not if) I fall.* Finally, lest I forget...*Thank you, Lord, for your love, help, guidance, and wisdom.* AMEN! Feel free to recite your own prayer. Just be sure to pray!

Choose the right time to start.

It is important to choose the right time frame for starting this journey. Valentine's Day is probably not the best day to start. Neither is your birthday. Find a two-to-three-week period on your calendar with the fewest social engagements. Surprisingly, the three-week stretch of time between Thanksgiving and Christmas was open for me to jump-start my weight loss. Because we were in the midst of the holiday season, however, some sweet treat was usually waiting for me in the office kitchen and calling my name, so I avoided that kitchen like the plague. By the time the holiday office party rolled around, I had lost the first eleven pounds. Needless to say, I realized I was on to something and was motivated to stick to my budding diet plan. Before the office party started, I filled up on water, and I served notice on my taste buds, stomach, and food addictions that I would be in the driver's seat that day. When the party started, I filled my plate with veggies and salad and ate those first. I then eyed the turkey, salmon, and other veggie dishes and indulged. By the time I had finished drinking the water and eating salad, raw veggies, tasty vegetable dishes, and lean meats, I was full and not tempted in the least by the heavy carbs or rich desserts.

Resist temptation—cheaters never prosper (or lose weight!)

As you shed the first ten pounds, you will discover temptation all around you. After all, no man or woman is an island. That thought is never truer than when you are trying to lose weight. This is because most of us do not eat alone. When time permits, we eat breakfast with family members. Most of the time, we gather with colleagues for lunch, and we usually eat dinner with family or out with friends after work. This is when things get sticky. Be prepared for well-meaning friends, family, and coworkers to tempt you with foods you should not eat. They just might pressure you to cheat, starting from day one. Cheating, however, will sabotage your attempt to lose the first ten pounds. Here's why: many of us are addicted to sugars, many food additives, and even trans fats. Losing the first ten is like going to food rehab. You have to cut some foods and beverages loose and actually go cold turkey to break those addictions. Cheating is like going to rehab for alcoholism but having a beer with your pizza while in rehab! We must break that craving. The first three to four weeks is *JustForMeDiet* rehab. If you successfully manage the first three to four weeks, you really are home free.

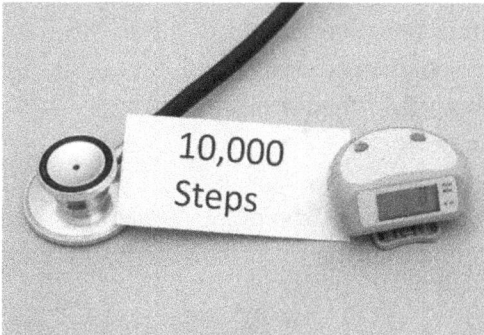

Aim for taking ten thousand steps per day.
You've heard the expression: "A body in motion tends to stay in motion." Conversely, "A body at rest stays at rest." Nothing could be truer. A body in motion is contracting muscles, revving metabolism, and regulating insulin, which is a key substance involved with weight loss. My doctor told me to buy a pedometer and to aim for taking ten thousand steps per day. Doing so was a nonnegotiable. From day one, I began wearing a pedometer to track my steps. We think we can estimate how many steps we are taking, but I realized that I underestimated that amount every single day. Therefore, I wear that pedometer faithfully, and I stagger my steps throughout the day. It serves no purpose to sit all day long and walk the ten thousand steps between 8:00–10:00 p.m. I clip the pedometer to my clothing first thing in the morning and monitor my progress throughout the day.

If possible, aim for two or three fifteen to twenty minute brisk walks per day, along with several smaller walk or movement breaks throughout the day in the place of the one hour walk. By all means, take the hour walk if your schedule permits, but be sure to break up the rest of the day with two to three minutes of walking, exercising in place, or some other movement every twenty to thirty minutes, if possible. Here are more reasons why walking every day should be a regular part of your life:[v]

BENEFITS OF WALKING:

1. Helps with weight loss
2. Helps reduce blood sugar
3. Helps prevent Alzheimer's disease and cognitive decline
4. Reduces the risk of heart attack and stroke
5. Reduces depression
6. Reduces belly fat
7. Improves your immune system
8. Lowers the risk of many cancers
9. Helps your body fight many existing cancers
10. Elevates your heart rate

Shall I go on? I think you get the point. While most people at age twenty or even thirty-five aren't thinking about chronic health conditions, you better believe that when you reach forty-five to fifty-five years of age, these conditions begin to hit close to home.

****

JUSTFORME TIP: *Walking Is Hard for Me Right Now.*
If walking is hard for you at this stage, don't worry; just start slowly and your strength and endurance will improve. Standing and walking or just moving every twenty to thirty minutes for just two minutes will make a huge difference to your weight and health. Consider water aerobics if your schedule permits, or invest in a mini trampoline for jumping and bouncing while you watch your favorite television show.
****

Weigh yourself every day.
This is like staring truth in the face every morning. Weigh yourself from day one, first thing in the morning after the first bathroom pit stop. Keep the scale in the same spot in the same room. *Wear nothing.* Trust me, I'd remove my hair if I could (some of us actually can, so take off the wig!). A digital scale is preferred because it delivers precision. It also shows your incremental progress. Every ounce lost is progress and is something to celebrate. Not only will weighing yourself every day reveal your progress but it will also let you see the impact of inactivity and certain foods on your weight—the good, the bad and the ugly, so you can make adjustments. Weighing yourself every day also lets you see "weight creep" as it happens. By the time your clothes become tight, you've already regained five pounds. So, be prepared to weigh yourself every day, pretty much for the foreseeable future.

Embrace the new you!
Believe it or not, as you lose the weight, your body will begin to change. The skin has a tendency to sag, particularly, when the weight loss is rapid. Those around you, even well-meaning family and friends, just might tell you that you look frail or sickly. Do not be alarmed. Again, those observations are based on years of seeing you and most of the people around us with the additional weight. Change is new and frightening. Reassure them and yourself that you are fine. Stay the course. Your skin will catch up to the rest of you. Remember, the BMI scale, along with your doctor's guidance, determine your target weight, not friends and family . . . or the mirror.

CHAPTER 3

My First Ten Steps

**Remember not the former things, nor consider the things of old.
Behold, I am doing a new thing; now it springs forth, do you not perceive it?
I will make a way in the wilderness and rivers in the desert.**
ISAIAH 43:18–19

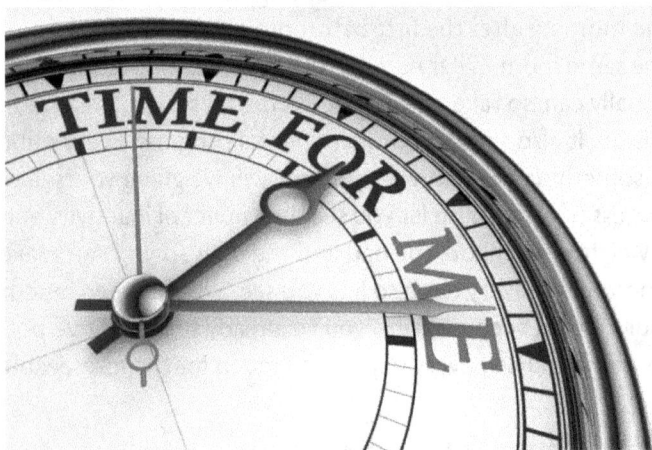

To bake a cake, you'll need to pick up a few ingredients from the grocery store. Likewise, your weight-loss success requires obtaining a few ingredients. The *JustForMeDiet* ingredient list starts with a calendar and a... marker. What? Why?

The calendar and the marker, or your cell phone, laptop, or iPad calendars will all ensure that you set aside the necessary time to plan and learn the *JustForMeDiet* and to begin implementation. Many of our goals and tasks remain unfinished because we have let life, our schedules, and even our health "happen to us" instead of taking the reins and being the one to call all the shots. We pencil ourselves in and are more than happy to erase the time we had set aside to care for our health and instead fill that time slot with a social event. I'm not saying we can't be sociable. It is a necessary part of life. But so is setting aside time to make sure that we are taking care of ourselves. If we don't, our bodies will stop us in our tracks. The marker is to ensure that you don't pencil yourself in anymore. Instead, you will designate your "me" time in black marker ink. Your health, happiness, longevity, and quality of life just might depend on that marker!

For me, the three biggest adjustments I had to make throughout this journey involved time, money, and overcoming family or social pressure:

1) Spending more time meal *and* snack planning, cooking with fresh ingredients, and evaluating nutrition labels and ingredient lists at the grocery store
2) Sacrificing some luxuries, such as eating out every week, to free up more resources for purchasing organic produce
3) Overcoming family and social pressure to eat what everyone else is eating

THE FIRST TEN STEPS

Schedule the "two-day."
To jump-start this exciting transition to a leaner and healthier you, you will need to reserve two full days to plan and implement your dietary changes. Let's keep it real—this means at least six to eight hours for each of the two days. Let's call it the "two-day." Remember that name. Take a Friday off and clear your Saturday. If you are not in a position to carve out two days, then you have a larger problem. Find your "two-day" and block it off. Do not, I repeat, do not sell your time to the lowest bidder. Once you have blocked off your "two-day," guard it with your life by learning to say no when the invitations come in. They will come in the form of e-vites to a bridal shower, baby shower, charity drive meeting, brunch, birthday party, book club meeting (*Finally, a Diet That's Just for Me!* is next month's book, right?), or committee meeting—and that's just Saturday morning! Just say...NO! If saying no is just too difficult a word for you, try these softer, kinder, gentler ways of saying the exact same thing:

I have a previous engagement (me!)...My schedule is booked (for me!) this weekend...Maybe next time...I have a deadline (to lose this weight), but give my regards to...

Get the picture? From this day forward, you must learn to *regularly* plan and schedule health promoting events. Cooking and meal preparations can no longer involve popping the frozen doohickey into the microwave so you and the kids can run back out the door. Mark your calendar to create your *JustForMeDiet* grocery list, your walks, doctor's visits, time for healthy meal preparation, and time to carve out physical activities throughout your day. These must all be priorities in your life. So let's explore what ingredients are on our two-day list:

The "two-day" list

✓ Buy, borrow or pull from storage your essential and ideal *JustForMeDiet* tools. Do not worry if you can't purchase these items all at once. These essential and ideal tools include:

Essential:

- Two pairs of walking shoes (one for work and one for home)
- A half-dozen pairs of footie socks
- A digital scale
- A good pedometer
- Two stainless-steel water bottles
- One hour every Sunday evening to plan the week's breakfasts and lunches, to pack your snacks, and to fill your water bottle
- An extra set of dishes (a plate, bowl, spoons, and forks) to keep at work with you
- *JustForMeDiet* partners

Ideal:

- A vegetable steamer
- An airtight bin to store your dishes and snacks at work
- A Ninja or Bullet blender (you might consider keeping one at work)
- A lunch crock-pot to reheat your leftovers *(available in retail stores)*

- Glass storage lunch and leftover containers to use in the microwave (I never, ever microwave or serve hot food on plastic or Styrofoam dishes or containers)
- A mini trampoline
- Hand weights
- Resistance bands
- A mini peddler
- A mini stair stepper
- An inexpensive tailor to alter your clothes after you begin to lose weight

****

JUSTFORME TIP: I Have No Way to Reheat Leftovers at Work.

No worries. If you can't or don't want to microwave your food, you can heat up your food in "lunch" crock-pots. Granted, your colleagues at work will be using the microwave and probably will think or even tell you that you've taken this health kick too far. I get that all the time. Ignore them and do your thing anyway. In addition, the JustForMeDiet provides several suggested no-cook lunches and snacks.

****

Weigh yourself.

The scale is not the enemy. Having a starting point allows us to measure our progress. There might be hurt feelings initially because it will tell you the truth, something we all try to avoid when it comes to our weight. Trust me, I understand completely! Over time, however, the scale will become your BFF (best friend forever).

Take your before and after pics.

I suggest that you have someone else take pics of you from every angle. You want before and after pics. Record where you are on the BMI scale and notate where you need to be. You also might want to take your body measurements to help track your progress.

Make a doctor's appointment, if possible.

You should know your blood pressure, cholesterol levels (both good and bad), A1C hemoglobin count, and vitamin and mineral levels (iron, B vitamins, D, calcium, and magnesium). Many, if not most, Americans are deficient in vitamin D *and* magnesium. Vitamin D deficiency is linked to obesity, diabetes and some cancers, among other health conditions. Do not be afraid to insist on having these tests done.

Track recent food and nutrient intake.

Record your meals, snacks, and beverages from the previous seven days. Ask members of your family to help you remember, if necessary. Look at your grocery receipts. This task helped me to see what I was eating. I took the time to look at the nutrient labels and realized I was burning money on foods containing trans fat, too many carbohydrates and high sugar content with little to no protein and fiber. My diet also lacked fresh fruits and vegetables. Only after looking at my seven-day record was I able to see what I was actually eating on a regular basis.

Inventory your food supply.

This exercise involves opening your cabinets and your refrigerator (include the secret stashes) and taking inventory of your foods. Categorize fresh fruits and vegetables, meats, breads and bread products, cereals, snacks, beverages, salad dressings, starches, and processed boxed food, such as processed mac and cheese, frozen meals, etc. Take a good, hard look at what is stocked in your kitchen. As you do so, take a few seconds per product to read the nutrition label, making a mental note of the sugars and carbohydrates, the fiber and protein content or lack thereof, the trans-fat content, as well as the ingredients. If you cannot see the ingredient list because the print is too small, or if you cannot pronounce most of the ingredients because they resemble terms you'd find in a chemistry book, or if the list of preservatives is longer than the Nile River, then you are picking up clues as to why we're obese and unhealthy.

TWO-MINUTE DRILL: STAND AND WALK!

Track recent exercise and movement history.

Record the last seven days' worth of exercise (when and how long): Weight lifting? Walking? Spinning class? Also, track all sedentary periods for the past seven days. You can track or record this information on the activity table found at Appendix C. For many of us, the table just might resemble something like this:

Time	Sun	Mon	Tue	Wed	Thu	Fri	Sat
7–8	Sleeping	Dressing, eating, commuting (mostly sitting)	Dressing, eating, commuting (mostly sitting)	Dressing, eating, commuting (mostly sitting)	Dressing, eating, commuting (mostly sitting)	Dressing, eating, commuting (mostly sitting)	Sleeping (Don't judge me!)
8–9	Dressing	Commuting or working at computer (sitting)	Commuting or working at computer (sitting)	Commuting or working at computer (sitting)	Commuting or working at computer (sitting)	Commuting or working at computer (sitting)	Relaxing (sitting) or preparing breakfast
9–12	Church, brunch (sitting)	Working at computer or in meetings (sitting)	Working at computer or in meetings (sitting)	Working at computer or in meetings (sitting)	Working at computer or in meetings (sitting)	Working at computer or in meetings (sitting)	Hair salon, kids' games, rehearsals (sitting)
12–1	Church (sitting)	Lunch w/friends (sitting)	Lunch at desk (sitting)	Lunch w/friends (sitting)	Lunch at desk (sitting)	Lunch w/friends (sitting)	Pizza after game (driving, sitting)
1–6	Cooking, TV, kids' games (sitting)	Working at computer or in meetings (sitting)	Working at computer or in meetings (sitting)	Working at computer or in meetings (sitting)	Working at computer or in meetings (sitting)	Working at computer or in meetings (sitting)	Errands, birthdays, meetings (sitting)
6–7	Cooking dinner	Commuting (sitting)	Spin class	Commuting (sitting)	Zumba class	Commuting (sitting)	Resting (Sitting)
7–9	TV time (sitting)	TV, homework time (sitting)	Commuting, TV time (sitting)	TV, homework time (sitting)	Commuting, homework (sitting)	church or TV time (sitting)	Out to dinner (driving, sitting)
9–11	Computer or TV time (sitting)	Computer or TV time (sitting or lying down)	Computer or TV time (sitting or lying down)	Computer or TV time (sitting or lying down)	Computer or TV time (sitting or lying down)	Computer or TV time (sitting or lying down)	Computer or movies (sitting)

Out of approximately 112 alert hours during the week, do you record less than six or seven non-sedentary hours? If so, use the blank table below the first table at Appendix C to revise your schedule to include walk or other "movement breaks" during every hour of the day.

Track the previous twelve months of eating (and drinking) out.

Similar to the way a financial planner requires you to track how your money is spent to identify the leaks, this exercise is designed to track where the weight is coming from. The problem is that most of us spend most of our time outside of our homes. As a result, many of our calories, carbohydrates, fats, and sugars are consumed *outside* of the home. This is the terrain we must conquer to lose the weight and keep it off. It starts by taking an honest assessment of what the damage is and where it is coming from.

Buy a calendar and notate for the previous twelve months all the office parties, birthday parties, celebration and church dinners, vacations, breakfast or other buffets (death by buffet), anniversary dinners, wedding receptions, funeral repasts, holiday meals, barbeques, office pizza parties, baby showers, eating with the lunch crowd, and going out to dinner. Include ordering-in days. Look at your credit-card statements for more detail. On some days, I ate out two or three times per day, three or more days per week. It turns out I ate out at least 30–40 percent of the 365 days of the year. I'm not suggesting we can't celebrate with family, friends, and colleagues, or eat on that ten-day Caribbean cruise (I could use a cruise right about now). Rather, we just need to dial it down a bit and plan how to handle those gatherings in advance.

Identify and record your nutritional needs.

I had to determine how many carbohydrates, proteins, fats, and fiber grams I needed to consume to lose the weight and maintain health. By the time we reach forty years of age, our metabolisms have slowed, and our cholesterol and blood sugar levels might be elevated. Most importantly, we are far less active than we were **in our twenties.** Therefore, our fuel needs are lower, meaning that our carbohydrate needs are not what they used to be. Nonetheless, we continue to eat carbs at the same levels we did when we were younger and more active. The resulting refined-carbohydrate *overload* with a protein, fiber, and healthy fat *deficiency*, along with being sedentary, were at the root of my inability to lose the dozens of pounds I gained over the years.

➢ Based on guidelines I discovered on the various health websites, including those at CDC, USDA, and at www.authoritynutrition.com ,[vi] I determined my average daily requirements of protein, carbohydrates, the fiber, fat, and sugar[vii] are as follows:

- Protein: 60–80 grams (derived from USDA recommendation that protein constitutes 10–25 percent of the total calorie intake. This range represents around 15 percent and 20 percent of a 1,700-calorie diet)
- Fiber: 22-25 grams
- Good fat: 40-60 grams (derived from USDA recommendation that good fat constitutes 20–35 percent of the total calorie intake. This range represents 20 percent and 30 percent of a 1,700-calorie diet)

- Carbs: 100 grams[viii] for the first few weeks since I was trying to lose weight; 130 grams thereafter)
- Sugar: 25 grams

Prepare to study nutrition labels, ingredient lists and serving sizes

Judge a product by its nutrition label and ingredient list. This process involves taking a field trip to the grocery store or to the product's website to familiarize yourself with nutrition labels of your favorite foods. I find it especially enjoyable to investigate the healthy-sounding labels to determine just how healthy (or not) the product really is. Look at the top of the label. Please, please pay attention to the "Serving Sizes." You need to know how many calories, proteins, fats, fibers, sugars, and carbohydrates are in the container itself. For example, the following label information is from a bottle of orange juice that provides the nutritional content *per serving*. According to the label, the juice contains 120 calories, twenty grams of sugar, and twenty-nine grams of carbs per serving. These numbers reflect one serving, but as you can see, the container actually contains *two* servings! And since you are likely to drink the whole bottle, you are downing fifty-six grams of sugar—over twice the sugar limit recommended for an adult woman.

➢ **Sample nutrition label**

Nutrition Facts		
Serving Size: 8 fl. oz (240 ml)		
Servings Per Container: 2		
Amount Per Serving		
Calories 120		
		% Daily Values
Total Fat 0g		
Saturated Fat 0g		0%
Trans Fat 0g		0%
Cholesterol 0g		0%
Sodium 0g		0%
Total Carbohydrate 29g		10%
Dietary Fiber 0g		0%
Sugars	28g	

> Over time, you will become a pro at studying the labels. For assistance, consult online nutrition calculators that will provide you with how many carbs, fats, sugars, and other nutrients are included in the foods and beverages you eat and drink. By the way, if the print on the label or list of ingredients is blended into the background of the wrapper, or is just too small for human eyes to read, which is increasingly the case, do not buy it. Send a message to the manufacturers informing them that you will no longer reward them for hiding their ingredients. Finally, as you find food and beverage items that are nutritionally acceptable to you, keep track of the brands so you never have to reinvent the wheel.

> **Examples from ingredient lists:**

If you reflect on your last trip to the grocery store, you probably will not recall having spent much time studying the ingredient list on many, if not most, of the processed foods you purchased. When you start reviewing those ingredient lists, you might run into these fellas:

> *Partially hydrogenated vegetable oil, citric acid, soybean oil, monosodium glutamate, maltodextrin, hydrolyzed vegetable protein, yeast extract, xanthan gum, sodium nitrate, sodium nitrite, high fructose corn syrup, soy lecithin, sucralose, natural flavors, spices, etc.*

I'll admit that when I used to go to the grocery store, I just purchased "food" without ever stopping to read the ingredient list or researching what those ingredients were doing to my body. I never made that leap because, well, I'm not really sure why. Is it that I was just too trusting? Is it that I just didn't have the time or didn't want to know? In any event, whatever impeded my curiosity in the past has been put out to pasture because it is time to know what we are eating and what we are feeding to our children. You don't have to believe me—just do your own research.

In fact, it's time for a homework break! Yes, you have homework (I bet you never thought you'd see the word "homework" in a diet book). Go to your kitchen cabinet and pull out a couple of boxed food products. Research some of those ingredients listed on the box and read what the research is telling us about those additives and preservatives. You'll discover that many of them are contributing to the weight, belly fat, fibroid tumors, gastrointestinal conditions, migraines, diabetes, dizziness, fatigue, arthritis, cancer (yes, cancer), and many other conditions. Class dismissed!

CHAPTER 4

Out with the Old!

All things are lawful, but not everything is helpful.
I CORINTHIANS 6:12

This next section involves taking a stroll into the kitchen armed with a trash basket—*a large one*. I had to toss everything that was causing me to gain and keep the weight on. I know, I know. How about just eating this food and never buying it again—waste not, want not, right? I'm sorry. You need to throw it out. The only way to move forward is to let go of the things that are part of your past. If you are like me (and if you are reading this book it's because you ARE like me and are willpower challenged), then you must admit that if the sugar-sweetened cereal, doughnuts, granola bars, cookies, juices, and soda are in the pantry or in the fridge, you will eat and drink them.

Before we go any further, I think it's only fair that you know why certain foods have to go. Throughout this book, you'll find discussions about lowering your blood sugar and avoiding sugar spikes and insulin resistance. In short, these conditions are linked to weight gain or weight loss, period. Let's talk about that for a quick moment—science class is in session for just a minute (my apologies). Then we'll get back to the fun stuff.

WARNING: SCIENCE LESSON...Insulin!

What is insulin anyway?
Insulin is a hormone made in the pancreas, an organ located behind the stomach. The pancreas makes and releases the insulin into the blood. Insulin plays a major role in metabolism—the way the body uses digested food for energy.

The digestive tract breaks down carbohydrates into glucose. Glucose is a form of sugar that enters the bloodstream. With the help of insulin, cells throughout the body absorb glucose and use it for energy. [ix]

Insulin's Role in Blood Glucose Control

According to the National Diabetes Information Clearinghouse (NDIC), when blood glucose levels rise after a meal, the pancreas releases insulin into the blood. Insulin and glucose then travel in the blood to cells throughout the body. Insulin helps muscle, fat, and liver cells absorb glucose from the bloodstream, lowering blood glucose levels. Insulin also stimulates the liver and muscle tissue to store excess glucose, and it lowers blood glucose levels by reducing glucose production in the liver. In a healthy person, these functions allow blood glucose and insulin levels to remain in the normal range.

What is insulin resistance?

Insulin resistance is a condition in which the body produces insulin but does not use it effectively.[x] Glucose builds up in the blood instead of being absorbed by the cells, leading to type 2 diabetes or prediabetes.

What does insulin resistance have to do with my weight?

NDIC explains that with insulin resistance, muscle, fat, and liver cells do not respond properly to insulin and thus cannot easily absorb glucose from the bloodstream. As a result, the body needs higher levels of insulin to help glucose enter cells. The pancreas tries to keep up with this increased demand for insulin by producing more. As long as the pancreas is able to produce enough insulin to overcome the insulin resistance, blood glucose levels stay in the healthy range. Over time, however, the pancreas fails to keep up with the body's increased need for insulin. When there's not enough insulin in the bloodstream, the muscles, fat, and liver cells can no longer absorb the glucose from the bloodstream, and the glucose builds up in the blood instead of being absorbed by the cells. This leads to type 2 diabetes or prediabetes. When your body can't absorb the glucose, **it is stored as fat.**[xi] Yes, it's a vicious cycle.

What causes insulin resistance?

Scientists, according to the NDIC, think the major contributors to insulin resistance are **excess weight** and **physical inactivity**. Let's look at both:

- **Excess Weight**

Obesity, especially excess fat around the waist, is a primary cause of insulin resistance. Belly fat produces hormones and other substances that can cause insulin resistance, high blood pressure, imbalanced cholesterol, and cardiovascular disease (CVD). Studies show that losing the weight can reduce insulin resistance and prevent or delay type 2 diabetes.

- **Physical Inactivity**

Many studies have shown that physical inactivity is associated with insulin resistance, often leading to type 2 diabetes. In the body, more glucose is used by muscle than other tissues. Normally, active muscles burn their stored glucose for energy and refill their reserves with glucose taken from the bloodstream, keeping blood glucose levels in balance.

Studies show that after exercising, muscles become more sensitive to insulin, reversing insulin resistance and lowering blood glucose levels. Exercise also helps muscles absorb more glucose without the need for insulin. The more muscle a body has, the more glucose it can burn to control blood glucose levels.

What helps to fix this?

Reducing the number of refined carbohydrate grams we eat is a good start toward losing the weight that contributes to insulin resistance.[xii] The more fiber we add to our carbohydrates, the less insulin resistance we have.[xiii] Fiber is like a sponge that soaks up the sugar. Fiber, and even protein and healthy fat, slow the fast and furious infusion of sugar or glucose into the bloodstream. Also, increasing the frequency of your physical activity, whether structured exercise classes, multiple walks per day, even daily "deskercises," will go a long way to reversing insulin resistance. Enough of the science! Class dismissed. So, let's look at what had to go…

OUT WITH THE OLD…

> **GROCERY LIST**

We go to the grocery store, grab the oversized cart, and start reaching for what we always buy: the same dairy products, the same meats, the same cereal boxes, the same snacks, the same frozen vegetables, the same packaged, frozen, or canned starches, the same condiments and salad dressings, and so on.

To implement the *JustForMeDiet*, throw away the old list and prepare to begin anew. I know change can be frightening, and no one really likes change. Change, however, is what we must do to meet our goals. From your "two-day" forward, be prepared to transition to new, tastier, fresher, and weight-loss-stimulating foods.

> ## ➤ INFLAMMATORY FOODS...IT STARTS WITH FAST FOOD!

What on earth is inflammatory food? I asked the same question. Inflammation is the body's immune response to illness or injury. It is a good thing, at least at first, but if it continues, it causes the body to break down and become diseased. Certain emotional conditions, such as depression, excessive and/or prolonged stress, and certain foods may result in the release of inflammatory chemicals (cortisol, for example) and hormones (estrogen) that, if released over a sustained period of time can cause disease and weight gain. Fast food, fried foods, processed and refined foods, and sugar are the worst offenders. You need to prepare to walk away from these "life shorteners" as discussed below.

Divorce French fries!
Inflammatory foods certainly include our old-time favorites. Breakfast biscuits, burgers, French fries, fried chicken, mashed potatoes, many canned soups, tacos, and even some salads because of the dressing are all suspect. I'll tell you why, although you already know why. These foods contain tons of trans fat, too much saturated fat, sodium (dangerously high amounts for those at risk for strokes), sugar, and empty carbohydrates. There really is no way around this. For me, these foods had to go. Oh, and don't think that a few extra minutes on the treadmill will offset the damage the fast-food frenzy most certainly will cause to our body's ability to manage glucose and process fat. Sadly, it simply doesn't work that way. I suppose that is why my doctor told me to go down to the courthouse and divorce French fries.

Fried food is inflammatory and contributes to disease.
As discussed, giving up fried foods really is nonnegotiable because of the inflammation it causes in the body. Inflammation is directly linked to cancer, diabetes, heart disease, depression, and belly fat. Without even considering the inflammatory impact to your body, just look at the nutritional damage caused by one fried chicken breast and fries:

- 440 calories, 27 grams of fat, and 110 mg of cholesterol
- Cajun-seasoned fries adds 770 calories with 41 grams of fat and 89 carbs

If you order the large orange soda, you add around three hundred extra calories, roughly eighty sugar grams, and eighty carb grams. The soda constitutes more than three days' worth of sugar. And you can forget the biscuit! I could have belly danced from now until the cows came home, but if I had not changed my diet and eliminated the sugar and the fast food and fried food fests, this book would not exist. By the way, many people ask me, "Jan, what's the healthiest oil for frying?" I used to rack my brain and waste time researching scores of conflicting information. Then I realized they were asking the wrong question. They should have asked: "Should I be frying food at all?" The answer is no. Aim to reduce or eliminate your food frying.

Now let's discuss what might be the largest inflammation maker out there: SUGAR!

➢ **SUGAR**

> ***It is not good to eat much honey.***
> **Proverbs 25:27**

Since the love of money is the root of all evil, one might say that the love of sugar is the root of all disease. I know that's a stretch, but I'm definitely in the ballpark. Sugar crashes the immune system, feeds cancer cells and bad bacteria in the gut, contributes to diabetes and cardiovascular disease, rots our teeth, and is poison to the eyes. No one disputes that we have a sugar problem in this country. In 2008, the average American consumed over seventy-five grams of sugar per day. That's three times the **twenty-five-gram limit** we're supposed to consume. [xiv]

Sugar is addictive.
According to recent studies, sugar might be as addictive as cocaine. Moment of silence…No wonder we seem to need a sugar fix from time to time. Just like cocaine, all it takes is one bite or one sip and our brains tell us, *give me more or you will suffer the consequences!* I know from personal experience that after just one grab out of the sugary breakfast cereal box, I cannot stop. One spoonful of ice cream, and we all know what happens next. Even after just one bite of the "organic and healthy cookie," and one day later, the empty cookie box is tossed into the trash can (meet the *real* Janessa!) So, I learned that the sugar battle is won at the grocery store. I stopped buying products with added sugar, period. The truth is that our intake of sugar and sugar products must be slashed drastically, and I

know more than anyone how hard that is. My taste buds like it sweet! So, we can at least eat "healthy sugars," right? Not so fast.

Are all sugars bad?

There is white sugar, brown sugar, confectioner's sugar, beet sugar, liquid sugar (sucrose), fructose, high fructose corn syrup, and others. Everyone is into raw sugar these days. It is widely believed that raw sugar, honey, agave nectar, molasses, and sugar alcohols are much healthier for you than bleached and processed sugar. And to some extent, that's true because many of those sweeteners, such as agave, coconut palm sugar, molasses, and brown rice syrup are known to have lower glycemic loads than processed and bleached white sugar, which is always a good thing. Sugar alcohols have little to no sugar grams. Because most sweeteners still contain sugar, however, I have learned to limit my intake of all of them. I choose the sugars with the lower glycemic load if I must choose, but I'll still keep the intake low. The truth is that when any of these sugars hits your bloodstream, *sugar is sugar*. That's because it all eventually becomes glucose. It may be called agave or raw sugar or honey, but we should always strive to minimize our use of all sweeteners.

Watch out for naturally occurring sugars.

Natural sugars are abundant in fruit juices and dried fruit. At about four grams of sugar per teaspoon, a twelve-ounce cranberry juice drink adds a whopping forty-eight grams of sugar to your body. How philanthropic! That twelve-ounce glass of orange juice? *Thirty-three grams* of blood-sugar-spiking sugar. That is too much sugar in one glass, which is why I had to discontinue the oversupply of the liquid orange. Will I eat an orange? Of course! Will I drink OJ anymore? No more than three to four ounces of the reduced sugar brands and never on an empty stomach!

Everyone is well aware of the obvious high-sugar sources, such as doughnuts, cakes, ice cream, candy bars, cookies, pies, and juicy drinks. Here are the hidden sources I thought you might want to know about:

Hidden sugars

- Raisins (29 g for just ¼ cup!) (For the longest time, I added a big chunk of raisins to my oatmeal or ate them in a baggie with nuts—no more!)
- Maple Syrup (28 g/2 tbsp.)
- Dried fruit and trail mixes (25–30 g/6 pieces)

- Sweetened yogurt (26 g/6 oz.)
- Many cold cereals (20–25 g/¾ cup)
- Coffee creamer (liquid: 18 g/3 tbsp.)
- Many salad dressings (14 g sugar/2 oz.)
- Some spaghetti sauces, including marinara sauce (13 g/serving)
- Jelly/Jams (8–13 g/tbsp.)
- Fat-free milk (12 g/cup)
- Baked beans (12 g/half cup) If you go back for seconds, you're a goner!
- Granola bars (8 g+)
- BBQ Sauce (8 g/2 tbsp.)
- Effervescent Vitamin C powder (5 g/packet)
- Vita C lozenges (5 g/drop) (I was devouring three or four at a time!)
- Cough drops (4 g/drop)
- Ketchup (4 g/tbsp.)

> **REFINED FOOD**

Refined and processed foods? You know—cookies, cakes, store-bought rolls and other bread products, cold cereals, crackers, pastas, and boxed pasta mixes, etc. These foods are thought to be inflammatory as well. If I had to guess, 90 percent of everything in your pantry or perched atop your refrigerator is *refined*, as was the case in my house. If it's in a box, the food is likely refined food products and is not food, in my humble opinion. These food products are higher in sugar, carbohydrates, sodium, questionable preservatives (such as monosodium glutamate, or MSG[xv]), additives, chemicals, and all sorts of stuff that we know little about unless you spend hundreds of hours researching what impact these ingredients have on our bodies. The list goes on. Refined foods are almost completely void of fiber, protein, or healthy fat, and yet, they are as American as apple pie and football. The *JustForMeDiet* goal is to minimize our intake of boxed, processed, or refined food.

> **HIGH-CARB, LOW-FIBER FOODS**

Only when I eliminated high-carb, low-fiber, low-protein snacks, beverages, and dishes did the weight begin to drop quickly. Consider this:

- A serving of white rice has forty-four grams of carbohydrates but less than one gram of fiber.

- A serving of spaghetti egg noodles has forty-two grams of carbohydrates, but only two and a half grams of fiber. (Who stops with one serving? Who in this country has one small serving of spaghetti noodles? When you add the garlic bread, you approach 100–120 grams of carbohydrates.)
- Just two twelve-inch tortillas have around one hundred–plus grams of carbohydrates, but only seven grams of fiber.
- Sixteen ounces of strawberry lemonade has sixty-nine grams of carbohydrates, but no fiber.

Trade, don't eliminate carbs.

I wanted to start discussing carbohydrates or "carbs" for short early in this book because they are so instrumental in weight loss and weight gain. Therefore, you'll see several chats here and there on the topic of carbs. This is not a "low-carb" or worse, a "no-carb" diet. I did not eliminate carbohydrates. Instead, I *switched* the type of carbohydrates I consumed, reduced the amount and, as discussed below, counted the carbs on a daily basis. The following are examples of my typical carb trades: Instead of cold cereal, I ate oatmeal nearly every day. Instead of white potatoes, I ate sweet potatoes. Instead of white rice, I ate brown rice, quinoa and other whole grains to meet my daily whole grain dietary requirement. Instead of two slices of refined bread or toast, I ate fruit or one slice of high-fiber whole grain bread. Instead of orange juice, I squeezed a lemon into a glass of water and added stevia or one teaspoon of coconut sugar. Instead of a bagel, I scrambled an egg with turkey sausage and ate grapes. Instead of egg noodle pasta, I ate one small serving of 100 percent whole grain pasta with no second helping; instead of sugar-sweetened yogurt, I reached for plain Greek yogurt and added my own fruit. At the end of week one, I had lost four pounds. The plan was working. At the end of week three, I had dropped eleven pounds. Let me tell you, I was astonished and motivated like never before!

Don't forget to count your carbs!

Again, we are accustomed to counting calories and fat. *Now you need to count your carbs and your sugars.* During the first few months, I ate around twenty-five carbs per meal with another twenty-five carbs for snacks. Likewise, I suggest you do the math up front. You then will know how you will divide your carbs by meals and snacks before you even take your first bite. As can be seen below, some foods were so carb-heavy that I had to toss them overboard to keep my diet boat afloat.

Castaways

I had to fire white potatoes, egg noodle pasta (distinguished from 100 percent whole-grain pasta), white rice, low-fiber breads, doughnuts, cakes, cookies, bagels, pies, mac and cheese, French fries, and...pizza. This change involved emptying my pantry and fridge, which at the outset of this journey consisted of frozen waffles, bagels, frozen diet meals (that are nuked in plastic!), processed pasta foods, sugary and soybean oil-filled salad dressings, high-carb/low-fiber self-proclaimed "healthy" breakfast cereal, crackers, juice drinks, chips, and cookies. They have been replaced. Instead, we now regularly prepare and eat sweet potatoes, whole grains, beans, and high-fiber/high-protein breads and snacks.

> **COLD CEREAL**

There are dozens of cold cereal brands on the market, and many promise nutrition and help with weight loss. Unfortunately, this is where we've judged a book by its cover. For decades, we have bought cold cereal because it is a quick and easy breakfast meal. Sadly, many cold cereals contribute to weight gain. Most deliver high carbohydrate but low fiber or protein content. Many are extremely high in sugar—even the "healthy" ones. For these reasons, I simply did not eat cold cereal during the first four months of the *JustForMeDiet* journey. I cut them loose!

Put your cold cereal brand to the test!

If you are at home, grab the cold cereal boxes and notice the carbohydrate-fiber ratio. Is it ten to one or two? Meaning: thirty grams of carbs, with three or four grams of fiber? Or is it forty-five grams of carbs with only one gram of fiber and seventeen grams of sugar per serving? Is the serving one cup or is it two-thirds of a cup? Yes, for some cold cereals, a serving is two-thirds of a cup. Really? I can eat that in one spoonful! It also means that the nutrition data is measured for a two-third-cup serving. If you have ever measured two-thirds of a cup of cereal, it might fill one-third of your bowl. Pour what constitutes a typical bowl of cereal into your bowl. Now measure the amount you poured and compare it to the nutrition label on the box to know how many carbs, sugars, fiber grams, etc. you are actually eating.

During the "two-day" outing at the grocery store, spend a few minutes in the cereal aisle and compare the carbohydrate, fiber, protein, and sugar content of all of your family's favorite cold cereals. What you see might shock you. Those cereals will not receive an honorable mention here. Only after I lost the first thirty pounds did I slowly incorporate high-fiber/protein/low-sugar cereals into my diet, and only on mornings when I had no time to prepare a meal.

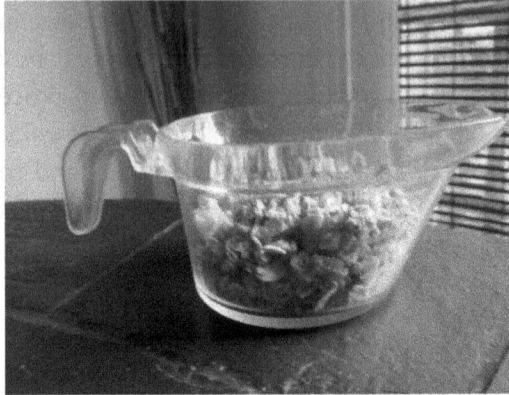

****
JUSTFORME TIP: My Kids Won't Eat Healthy Cereal.
Let them be a part of the process of selecting healthy alternatives. For example, let them taste your top-five choices, and ultimately decide which cereals are best for you and your family. If that doesn't work, negotiation and bribery usually work with most kids.
****

> **BREAD: THE STAFF OF LIFE...OR IS IT?**

Man shall not live by bread alone...
Matthew 4:4

That's because it needs butter, right? Wrong! I know I am moving into sacred-cow pasture here. Bread, after all, is the staff of life, right? This item has special meaning for me (a recovering breadaholic), so it is with care, empathy, and compassion that I gently approach this next food item. When I tell a friend who wants to know how I lost the weight to give up bread, they look the other way, sigh, or think to themselves, *Janessa has lost her mind*, particularly when I suggest that "Grapes are the new toast," or to stop eating sandwiches. It's un-American. Toast, biscuits, subs, other rolls, and sandwiches have become staples for breakfast, lunch, and dinner food. When you go to restaurants, bread is usually the first thing brought out to you. And we look forward to that hot bread—whether with honey butter or with pesto or some other olive oil concoction—we want it! Gotta have it! Give up my bread? Really? That's exactly what I thought when my doctor told me to back away from the bread.

Are you asking me to give up sandwiches?

During my forty-five-pound weight-loss journey, eliminating sandwiches for lunch was the best thing since sliced bread! Seriously, I know I'm moving into sensitive terrain—sandwiches in America, but I'm in the witness-protection program. Trust me, I was raised on sandwiches. But a funny thing happened during my separation from most bread products—the weight came off! Now, I have around three to four slices per week, and that's it. While we need the whole grains on a daily basis, we must not overdose on bread, crackers, rolls, cereals, subs and the like. There are many other ways – eating oatmeal, brown rice, quinoa, barley, buckwheat, and organic corn - to meet our whole grain dietary requirements. Again, many bread products contain too many carbs without the accompanying fiber and protein. A good carbohydrate/fiber ratio should be one to two grams of fiber for every ten grams of carbohydrates. Breads with one gram of fiber and one gram of protein offer *nothing but carbs*. The more protein and fiber per slice, the more filled you are, and for longer periods of time.

Also, sugar spikes are reduced when you include more fiber and protein in your bread products. If your bread, rolls, bagels, cereal, and crackers can't deliver the fiber, I suggest that you find some brands that do. When I do buy bread, I make sure that the brand delivers three to six grams of fiber and three to six grams of protein *per slice*. Otherwise, it's a no-go. Equally important to me is that the bread, buns, sub and dinner rolls, biscuits, and bagels have no soybean oil added, unless it is organic. If the oil is not organic or the bottle doesn't display the non-GMO (non genetically-modified) label, then I presume that the soybean oil is genetically modified.

What's in a label?

If you are at home, stop reading right now and grab your store-bought bread. Read the nutrition label. Unless the bread you are eating has a healthy dose of fiber and protein, you might be heading for the carb overload we're trying to eliminate from your diet. It does not matter that the bread is named: *The Staff of Life, Manna from Heaven, Healthy, Whole, 998 Grain, Super Food Bread,* or *Made by Grandma Bread.* You *must* read the nutrition label to see what's really in it. This "Read the nutrition label" rule goes for all the foods you purchase, beginning today, for the rest of your life!

When we buy bread, it's organic.

After you have read the nutrition label on your bread packaging, read the ingredient list and see if you see "soybean oil" or "soy lecithin." Do not be surprised when you do. One day, I spent about thirty minutes in the bread aisle of a local supermarket looking for bread that did not have soybean oil. I could not find one single brand until I searched in the organic aisle. The majority of breads are made with soybean oil. Although the packaging does not label the soybean oil as genetically modified, or GMO, I presume so, since at least ninety percent of all soybean oil used in this country is currently GMO.

****

JUSTFORME TIP: *Restaurant Strategy*
> *Just say no to bread. Not gonna happen?*
> *Okay, well, at least ask the server to bring your salad*
> *before he brings the bread!*

****

➤ OBESOGENS

There's that word again. I wonder if it's in the dictionary yet. Let me check. I'll get back to you...I just checked. It's not there yet. Well, rest assured, it will be soon. These are the chemicals and other things that do their part to make us fat. Hence, the "obeso" part of the word. Your mission, should you decide to accept it, is to create your own master obesogen list [BPA plastic water bottles, foods with MSG or added hormones, shampoo with parabens, and so on] to determine what you need to eliminate to give yourself a fighting chance at not just weight loss but improved overall health. Your homework assignment for the evening is to spend twenty minutes researching these search terms: *obesogens and obesity.* Be informed and make your own choice. You will find a preview of some of those obesogens in Chapter 11. Share what you find with your loved ones even as you strive to eliminate the obesogens in your life.

➤ FRUIT JUICE AND JUICE DRINKS

In chapter 9, we explore what's wrong with fruit juice and juice drinks. Suffice it to say that the nutritional benefit they bring to the table is often offset by their damaging high sugar (albeit "natural" sugar) content. Leave them at the grocery store. Instead of drinking the juice, eat the fruit.

➤ OVERCOOKED VEGETABLES

There isn't a person reading this book who hasn't overcooked their vegetables. We usually boil them, don't we? After all, that's what the frozen package instructs us to do. You know, "Bring the water to a boil, and put the frozen vegetables in the boiling water. Cover and boil for five to seven minutes. Drain and serve." Then, when we serve the vegetables, the water in the pot is the color of the vegetables. Of course, when it's time to wash the dishes we pour that water out. Well, guess what—there went the vitamins and other nutrients right down the drain! Look, if you're not going to reap the benefit of the vegetables, why pay all that money? We finally learned to sauté, roast, or steam our vegetables. Yes, buy a steamer. Alternatively, this is one of those times when you *can* drink the water! Yes, I know it's green.

CHAPTER 5

In with the New!

Old things are passed away, behold all things are new!
2 CORINTHIANS 5:17

Now that you have parted with some of the old ways and old foods, let's explore suggestions and alternatives that will launch the weight loss success you desire. Applying the "healthy trinity" concept is one of those suggestions.

THE HEALTHY TRINITY

In this section, I identify three macronutrients[xvi]: protein, fiber, and healthy fat that your meals *and snacks* should include if possible. I don't need to tell you to include carbohydrates (carbs) because you already will. We always do. Most meals and snacks on the market and in our kitchens are heavily "carbed." This section introduces us to the macronutrients that we have ignored at great cost to our health and body sizes.

1. THE POWER IS IN THE PROTEIN

In his article, "Protein Intake – How Much Should You Eat Per Day?" Kris Gunnars, at Authority Nutrition (http://authoritynutrition.com/how-much-protein-per-day/), states that "*Quite possibly the most important contribution of protein to weight loss is its ability to reduce appetite and cause a spontaneous reduction in calorie intake. Protein is much more satiating than both fat and carbs.*" The same article revealed that, in one study, women who increased protein intake to 30 percent of calories ended up eating 441 fewer calories per day. They also lost eleven pounds in twelve weeks, just by *adding* more protein to their diet.

Protein, particularly when eaten in the morning, helped my energy reserves to last longer than when I ate high-carb/low-protein-only breakfasts. I was far less hungry and ate less when I reached my protein requirements. When I ate less...guess what? I LOST WEIGHT!! I learned to cook with more plant and fish protein, lean and skinless chicken, and very lean red meat on a very limited basis. We eat beef liver from time to time because of the iron content. Note: this is *not* a high-protein diet. Rather, the goal is to meet my regular daily requirement of protein, a goal I used to miss because I ate way too many carbohydrates and never gave counting protein grams a second thought. Again, I didn't go crazy with protein shakes or smoothies. I accomplished the required protein intake by planning well-balanced meals and snacks.

How much protein should we eat?

The CDC recommends that 10–35 percent of our daily calories come from protein.[xvii] Each gram of protein contains four calories. Naturally, the most sedentary among us or those incapable of any physical activity should aim for the 10 percent range. Hopefully, if you are reading this book, you will not remain sedentary. Indeed, the more active you are, the closer to the middle or higher end of the range you should be. I aim for obtaining 15 –20 percent of my calories from protein because I am reasonably active. Since I consume around 1700 -1800 calories per day (more on some days; rarely less), the CDC formula results in a range of about 60-85 grams of protein per day. The more active I am on any given day, the more protein I will eat. I rarely eat more than eighty grams, however. Below I show you how I calculated my range of around 60-85 grams of protein per day:

FORMULA TO CALCULATE PROTEIN INTAKE:

1700 (calories eaten) x 15 % (of calories from protein) = 255 / 4 (calories per protein gram)

= 63 protein grams per day

OR

1700 (calories eaten) x 20 % (of calories from protein) = 340 / 4 (calories per protein gram)

= 85 protein grams per day

Your age, level of physical activity and muscle mass all should be considered when determining how many protein grams you should consume per day. Before I lost the weight, I realized I wasn't eating enough protein. Once I increased my protein intake, the weight began to fall off. Most women over the age of forty probably should aim for eating 10-15 percent of their calories from protein.

I always have protein with breakfast.

When I consume about fifteen grams of protein with breakfast, I am full and have no cravings of any kind for the rest of the morning. Hunger slowly begins to stir around 1:00 p.m. After evaluating my prior eating habits, I discovered that I did not consume even forty protein grams per day. When I did, those protein grams came late in the day, rather than in the first part of the day when I needed them most. Breakfast often consisted of an overabundance of carbohydrates with very little protein or fiber. That practice led to binges and heavy snacking. I experienced sugar spikes, which slowed my metabolism. I was hungrier sooner than if I had consumed protein with breakfast. I learned that the morning MUST include that healthy dose of protein. Below are examples of good protein sources for a variety of meals and snacks:

- 4 ounces lean sirloin steak — 24-30 g
- One half chicken breast (skinless/boneless) — 27 g
- 4 ounces fish or seafood (salmon, haddock, whiting, shrimp, etc.) — 22-27 g
- 1 cup plain nonfat Greek yogurt — 23 g
- 4 ounces lean turkey meat — 18 g
- 1 cup cooked lentils — 18 g
- 1 cup cooked lima, kidney or black beans — 15 g
- 1 cup plain nonfat yogurt — 12 g
- 1/4 cup of peanuts — 10 g
- 1 slice nonfat mozzarella cheese — 9 g
- 1 slice Swiss cheese — 8 g
- 1 egg — 6 g
- 2 tbsp. chia seeds — 4.7g
- 7 walnuts — 4 g

****

JUSTFORME TIP: What If I Don't Eat Red Meat or Poultry?

Too bad. Just kidding! In many cultures, fish is all the "meat" the citizens eat, and they have longer life expectancies and lower rates of cancer and heart disease than Americans. Beans and lentils contain a very healthy dose of protein and fiber. Have them two to three times per week. Also, if you are not allergic to nuts, they are a great weapon in your weight-loss arsenal and a great meat substitute. Most nuts are high in healthy fat and have a reasonable portion of protein. They can be incorporated into all meals and snacks. Occasionally, I add a few ounces of almond milk to my coffee and smoothies. Chia seeds also are loaded with protein and fiber.

****

Quick No-Cook-Any-Meal Protein Ideas

Here are some *JustForMeDiet* any-meal favorites for ensuring I get protein and other great nutrients on the fly:

Yogurt

Plain nonfat regular and Greek yogurts are very nutritious yogurts, useful for breakfast, lunch, snacks, and dessert, and both types of yogurt were a huge part of my weight-loss success. The trick is to select from the dizzying choices of yogurts and to eliminate the heavily sugared yogurts derived from cows that were given growth hormones and antibiotics. I usually opt for the organic non-fat plain and nonfat Greek yogurts with the lowest sugar content. Milk products have natural sugars, so the last thing you need are milk products with more sugar added. It took me a while to figure out that my organic, fat-free, lactose-free (yes, I know, TMI!) milk carried with it twelve grams of sugar per cup, thus earning a spot on the coveted "hidden sugars" list. Therefore, I incorporated almond milk into my milk repertoire. I also began to choose organic yogurt to ensure that my yogurt was not derived from cows that had been given artificial growth hormones or antibiotics. Because Greek yogurt contains nearly twice the protein of regular nonfat yogurt, my personal serving size is limited to six ounces.

By adding almonds or walnuts, berries, and one to two tablespoons of toasted oats, you can create a concoction that works for breakfast, lunch, snack, and dessert.

Beans and other legumes

Beans and other legumes, such as lentils and peas, are a great source of protein, fiber, iron, and other nutrients that can satisfy and nourish you at the same time. Even when I was younger, my father regularly served kidney beans over grits with breakfast. Yes, it was tough parting with grits during my forty-five-pound weight-loss odyssey. I'll try to move on. I buy canned black beans (BPA-free cans) and lentils. You can pour them over salad. Eat them with brown rice, quinoa, alongside guacamole, with eggs, or in a bowl with some chopped cilantro (okay, does this sentence sound like something out of a Dr. Seuss book?). Anyway, beans were non-negotiable in my weight-loss quest. They contain *good* carbohydrates. We eat black beans, kidney beans, white beans, even lima beans (loaded in iron). I admit that incorporating beans at lunch is a bit easier than forcing the "bean-bigoted" men in my house to accept beans as a substitute for meat at dinnertime, but they're getting there. Lentils cannot be beat for their high protein, fiber and iron content.

Smoothies (homemade, please!)

With homemade smoothies, *you* control the sugar content and can include whatever you want to include. I prepare my smoothies with different ingredients each time, and my protein sources range from a handful of nuts to yogurt, chia seeds, wheat germ, organic low-fat milk, almond milk, or whey protein powder if the smoothie is replacing a meal.

Tuna salad

This dish is easy to prepare and very good to the taste buds. I had many tuna lunches as I lost the weight, but I realized I needed to cut back because tuna contains mercury. Chunk Light tuna has lower mercury amounts than others. I still eat tuna once or twice per month. I now open a BPA-free can of tuna, add diced red onions diced apples (yes, apples!), cilantro, pepper, organic or soy-free mayo (one to two tablespoons) and some lemon juice. You can eat them with carrots, bell peppers or organic high-fiber crackers.

Chia seeds added to soups, salads, beans, smoothies and chili

Chia seeds are a great source of protein, fiber, and other nutrients. You can sprinkle them on oatmeal, beans, stews, and blend two tablespoons into your home-made smoothies, oatmeal, yogurt, or chili.

Some protein bars

Protein bars contain a healthy dose of protein (nine to twelve grams or more per bar), and many are a good source of fiber as well. Even when buying organic bars, I reach for the ones that contain less than twenty grams of sugar. If I cannot find bars that are organic, I purchase bars that are USDA or non-GMO certified.

2. FIBER IS YOUR FRIEND

Eating enough fiber is an absolute must if you plan on losing weight. You need to do the math to make sure you are eating the required amount. The daily requirement of fiber for women under the age of fifty is around twenty-five grams/day for women and around thirty-five to forty grams/day for men under the age of fifty. For some reason, that number decreases slightly once we turn fifty years old. Great sources of fiber include beans, oatmeal, buckwheat and other whole grains, many fresh or frozen fruits, and veggies such as broccoli, cucumber, avocado, artichoke, sweet corn, and sweet potatoes. In fact, one cup of black beans has around twelve grams of fiber!

Not all fiber is created equal

There are two types of fiber: soluble fiber and insoluble fiber. Let's take a look at each type:

Soluble fiber "attracts water and forms a gel which slows down digestion. . . [It] delays the emptying of your stomach and makes you feel full, which helps control weight. Slower stomach emptying should have a beneficial effect on insulin sensitivity, which may help control diabetes."[xviii] Soluble fiber can also help lower LDL ("bad") blood cholesterol by interfering with the absorption of dietary cholesterol. (Finally, a good "side effect!")

- **Sources of soluble fiber:** oatmeal, oat cereal, lentils, apples, oranges, pears, oat bran, strawberries, nuts, flaxseeds, chia seeds, beans, dried peas, blueberries, cucumbers, celery, and carrots.

Insoluble fibers are "gut-healthy fiber because they have a laxative effect and add bulk to the diet, helping prevent constipation. These fibers do not dissolve in water, so they pass through the gastrointestinal tract relatively intact, and speed up the passage of food and waste through your gut. Insoluble fibers are mainly found in whole grains and vegetables."[xix] You've heard of probiotics, right? Well, insoluble fibers are "prebiotics" that feed the probiotics to help keep your gut healthy. Healthy gut = healthy immune system. Accordingly, both types of fiber have an important role in our digestion, overall health, and weight loss goals.

- **Sources of insoluble fiber:** whole wheat, whole grains, wheat bran, corn bran, seeds, nuts, barley, couscous, brown rice, bulgur, zucchini, celery, broccoli, cabbage, onions, tomatoes, carrots, cucumbers, green beans, dark leafy vegetables, raisins, grapes, fruit, and root vegetable skins.

If the fiber content in your meals and snacks aren't adding up to the minimum daily amount, go back to the drawing board. Black beans with salsa, guacamole (guaca) and a few organic tortilla chips can comprise a quick and easy lunch or dinner, and you obtain nearly *all* of your fiber for the day—ten grams from the guaca and twelve grams from the beans. Are you catching on? Glad to hear! The Department of Agriculture[xx] graciously provided the fiber content for most of the following foods:

- 1 cup lentils   16 g
- 1 cup lima beans   13 g
- 1 cup black beans   12 g
- 1 cup kidney beans   11 g
- 2 tbsp. chia seeds   10 g
- 1 avocado   10 g
- 1/2 cup dry roasted peanuts   9 g
- 1/2 cup cooked green peas   9 g
- 1 cup raspberries   8 g
- 1 cup blackberries   8 g
- 1/2 cup corn (organic only)   6 g
- 1 slice high-fiber bread   6 g
- 1 med. size apple w/peel   4 g
- 1 small sweet potato   4 g
- 1 cup oatmeal   4 g
- 1 medium orange   3 g

The above list is by no means exhaustive, but it's a start. Select your favorites for stocking in your refrigerator, pantry, car, and office, so that when it's mealtime, or when you get hungry, you'll have what you need to curb the hunger. The fiber will fill you and keep you full. Going forward, your carbohydrates must have a partner—fiber and/or protein. When your carbs have their dance partner, there will be no need to fall off the wagon.

Whole Grains
Whole grains are a great source of fiber, protein and many other nutrients. The dietary guideline for whole grains, found at www.choosemyplate.gov, recommends

that we eat at least *five to six ounces of grains per day with at least three of those ounces in the form of whole grains.* One slice (1 ounce) of whole-grain bread, 1/2 cup brown rice, and 1/2 cup of oatmeal, each, is equivalent to three ounces of whole grains. In fact, a 2000-calorie diet requires at least four ounces of whole grains per day. Sadly, most breads and bread products, pastas, white rice, and crackers are made with grains that have been stripped of their fiber. Bakers, take note of this factoid: One cup of white flour has nearly 500 calories and only 1.6 grams of fiber, whereas one cup of whole wheat flour has only 384 calories with over 14 grams of fiber.

Popular members of the whole grain family include: whole wheat, quinoa, buckwheat, barley, bulgur, corn, kamut, millet, oats, rice (brown, black and red), rye, and wild rice. These whole grains are loaded in nutrients and fiber and, therefore, must be a part of your daily diet. The *JustForMeDiet* incorporates several of these whole grains, including oats, corn, whole wheat (high fiber bread), quinoa, and brown rice. Since I have challenged you to incorporate new foods into your diet, I will do the same by adding some of the other whole grains listed here. I'll start with buckwheat and millet, and I'll work my way to kamut and bulgur. Let's compare notes later on. It's later . . . I recently ate buckwheat groats (don't ask – actually, they are the hulled kernels) as a hot cereal. Not bad.

Note: While I obtained my daily grain requirement, including the right amount of whole grains, I did not eat *more* than the recommended daily amount. Again, eating too many servings of carbohydrates hinders your weight loss efforts.

3. FIGHT FAT WITH...*FAT!*

What? Is she serious, you may ask. Yes, we've been programmed to believe that all fat is bad. Fat is a cruel word used by kids on the playground. Trying to rid your body of *fat* is why you're reading this book. So how on earth can I fight fat with fat? That's like sleeping with the enemy, right? Not exactly. There are different types of fat—some good and some bad. Fat is a major source of energy and it helps the body absorb vitamins. It helps to lower the glycemic load and thus minimizes fat storage. Therefore, it is important to obtain the recommended daily requirement.

How much fat should we eat?
According to the CDC, we should consume 20–35 percent of our total calorie intake from fat. Each fat gram contains 9 calories. Therefore, with that same 1700

calorie diet, at *20 percent* of the calories, the CDC's formula results in a fat intake of 38 fat grams. At *30 percent* of the calories, the recommended fat intake is 57 fat grams. Surprised? Don't be. See the calculation below.

FORMULA TO CALCULATE FAT INTAKE:

1700 (calories eaten) x 20 % (of calories from fat) = 340 / 9 (calories per fat gram)

= 38 fat grams per day

OR

1700 (calories eaten) x 30 % (of calories from fat) = 510 / 9 (calories per fat gram)

= 57 fat grams per day

As can be seen, for a 1700 calorie diet, the most sedentary of us should limit our fat intake to 38 grams per day. If you are not sedentary or if you eat more than 1700 calories per day, you might need more fat in your diet. Below is a handy dandy chart from www.health.gov that sets forth the total fat limits for varying calorie levels:

MAXIMUM TOTAL FAT INTAKE AT DIFFERENT CALORIE LEVELS

Calories	1600	2,200	2,800
Total fat (grams)	53	73	93

Note: There is a variation between the recommendation provided by the CDC and the chart provided from www.health.gov. Your doctor should weigh in on what your fat range should be.

For me, a middle-aged woman with a fair amount of daily physical activity (well, at least from mid-March through mid-November) and a typical range of 1700 – 1800 calories eaten per day, my fat gram range is around fifty to sixty grams of fat. If you have a totally fat-free diet, you are depriving yourself of a macronutrient that will help you lose weight and absorb the vitamins from your food. The trick is to switch fats. Eat the good fats and lose the bad fats. Let's take a look at which is which:

GOOD FAT: Omega-3 (fish such as salmon, mackerel, herring, tuna, rainbow trout, walnuts, flaxseed, and flaxseed oil), monounsaturated and polyunsaturated fats (avocado, almonds, and other nuts and seeds, peanuts and peanut butter, olives and olive oil)

- o Supplies energy for body cells
- o Provides a protective layer around essential organs and nerves
- o Forms a structural component of brain tissue
- o Helps the body absorb and transport certain nutrients
- o Helps maintain normal heart function
- o Supplies essential fatty acids that the body can't make by itself[xxi]

Not only that, but the CDC Report, "Can Lifestyle Modifications Using Therapeutic Lifestyle Changes (TLC) Reduce Weight and the Risk for Chronic Disease?" (Research to Practice Series, No. 7, National Center for Chronic Disease Prevention and Health Promotion, Division of Nutrition, Physical Activity, and Obesity) recommends actually *increasing* the amount of monounsaturated and polyunsaturated fats from the U.S.'s estimated mean daily consumption as part of that lifestyle modification.

Are you eating enough good fat?

The TLC Recommendation for monounsaturated fats (ex. olive oil) is to increase our consumption from the current 12 percent mean to 20 percent of our total calorie intake, and to increase our consumption of polyunsaturated fats (ex. walnuts, seeds, flaxseed, salmon, tuna and mackerel) from the current 6 percent mean to 10 percent of our total calorie intake, for a total of 30 percent of our total calorie intake. Doing so will help reduce inflammation and insulin resistance - conditions that contribute to weight gain. Also, if your body is receiving the nutrients in needs, which the "healthy" fat then will transport and help your body absorb, your cravings should diminish.

Fat also gives us a feeling of fullness, thus curbing the appetite. Grandma was right! It actually works to calm the savage beast that controlled me—my appetite! So, as you can see, eliminating *all* fat from your diet is in fact sabotaging your weight-loss efforts. Moment of silence...

The typical range for most middle-aged individuals is from forty-five to seventy-five grams of good fat per day. Check with a nutritionist or doctor to determine what should be your fat consumption or range. I typically consume fats found in nuts, avocados, sunflower, sesame and pumpkin seeds, olive and coconut oil, and fatty fish such as tuna,[xxii] salmon (wild caught,[xxiii] if possible), mackerel, sardines, and trout. My regulars are olive oil, nuts, avocados, and Omega-3 fatty acids found in oily fish, flaxseed, and walnuts. Finally, I try not to exceed sixty grams per day. Even too much of a good thing is not so good, which is why meal planning is so important. You do the math.

SOURCES OF GOOD FAT (See www.choosemyplate.gov and product packaging)

- 14 walnut halves   18 g
- 2 tbsp. peanut butter   16 g
- 1 tbsp. coconut oil   14 g
- 1 tbsp. olive oil   14 g
- 4 ounces salmon, wild   12 g
  caught (cooked fillet)
- 1/2 avocado   10.5 g
- 10 almonds   7 g
- 2 ounces chunk lite tuna   4.5 g
- packed in oil, drained

BAD FAT: Trans fat and too much saturated fat round out this category. The discussion below explains why.

Trans fat: Trans fat is the clear winner as the bad-fat villain, hands down. According to the CDC, naturally occurring trans fat is found in small amounts in the fatty parts of meat and dairy products. Artificial trans fat comes from foods that contain partially hydrogenated oil and is formed when hydrogen is added to liquid oil, which turns it into solid fat. Often, food manufacturers use artificial trans fat in food products because it is inexpensive and it increases the food's shelf life, stability, and texture. You will find trans fat in most fast-food products and in many processed or refined foods.[xxiv]

Too much saturated fat: Some saturated fat is good for you, but we must keep our saturated fat intake in check. The site www.Health.gov suggests we limit saturated fat to no more than 33 percent of our total fat intake per day. Coconut oil is high in saturated fat. Again, the key is moderation and ensuring that your saturated fat consumption does not exceed 33 percent of your daily fat intake as recommended by health officials. During my weight loss journey, my goal was to consume my fat grams in the form of Omega-3 fats, as well as the monounsaturated and polyunsaturated fats, and to limit the saturated fat accordingly. By doing so, the weight loss was successful. Below are eye-popping examples of fat-filled foods that do far more harm than good:

BAD TRANS OR OVERLY SATURATED FAT FOODS

- 1 southwest chicken salad   90 g (Can you believe this one from a popular restaurant chain?)
- 1 serving seafood linguine   50 g
- 1 chicken pot pie   41 g (didn't see that one coming, did ya?)
- 1 quesadilla   27 g
- 1 double cheeseburger   26 g
- 1 fried chicken breast   20 g
- 1 serving large fries   24 g
- 1 cup ice cream   24 g
- 1 slice deep-dish pizza   20 g

Note: Restaurant and grocery store portion sizes vary but the above selections are examples from restaurant dishes or store bought products. Watch those restaurant "salads." They are not your friends!

****

JUSTFORME TIP: I'm Allergic to Nuts.
> *If you are allergic to nuts, you are not alone. Fortunately, there are several other sources of good fats to consume, such as salmon, cod, olive oil, avocado, eggs, and even coconut oil or butter in moderation.*

****

NEW TASTES TO FLAVOR YOUR FOOD!

So, what good is all that protein, fat, and fiber if my food doesn't taste good? Well, it still can. Actually, it will taste better than ever. As Americans, we've judged flavor based on how sweet, salty, or fat our food tastes. Since I told you what I left behind, let me tell you what I welcomed to the fold.

Develop a taste for the savory.

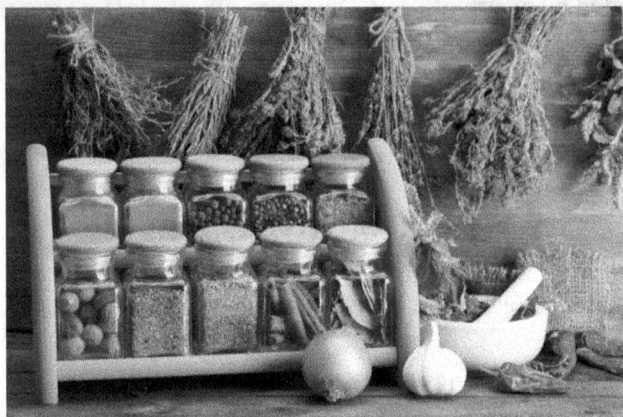

Over the past few years, I have trained my taste buds to move away from the salty and sugary-sweet taste to the savory, spicy, herbal, minty, citrusy, and nutty. I cook with rosemary (the memory herb), basil, oregano, dill, cilantro (it helps clear mercury out of the body), chives, sage, thyme, and many other herbs that flavor all of our food. I actually grow them...in the backyard...on the deck...in the kitchen...in the living room...in the basement...wherever I can.

Try cinnamon, nutmeg, turmeric, spice extracts, and fruit such as apples, dates, and bananas as alternatives to refined sugar.
Cinnamon is believed to help lower blood-sugar levels. I use cinnamon and nutmeg in oatmeal, sautéed apples, sweet potato dishes, and even in chili. Dates are good sweeteners with a low glycemic load. I add turmeric to scrambled eggs, soups, chili, beans, and marinades. It is used in many Indian and West Indian dishes (yummy!).

Switch to small amounts of coconut sugar, raw honey, and organic stevia.
Instead of using processed white sugar to sweeten my foods and beverages, I now use a teaspoon of coconut sugar or honey, or one or two packets of organic stevia in my coffee, tea, lemonade, oatmeal and smoothies. I even bake with stevia. You might not need any sweetener at all. When I add cinnamon to my coffee, I can do without sweeteners. By this time next year, I hope to drink my coffee without any type of sweetener. I'll let you know how that works out. At least for now, instead of four teaspoons of refined sugar in my coffee (the old me), I use these great alternatives, and I occasionally add two ounces of low fat

organic milk or unsweetened almond milk, which gives the coffee a nutty flavor. It took some getting used to, but I now like the taste. I choose health over sugar.

It may take you a couple of weeks to adjust to less sugar or no sugar, but let's face it - our sugar tolerance is much too high. Even our sweet tooth has diabetes! We really need to dial down the sweet teeth—way down. Learn to adjust to a lower sweet threshold. Although these alternative products simply don't taste the same as refined white sugar, your health—maybe even your life—may depend on learning a healthier way.

****

JUSTFORME TIP: *Stevia Upsets My Stomach.*
If stevia upsets your stomach, use honey or coconut sugar because of their low glycemic index. Coconut sugar contains B vitamins and really does taste good!
****

Fruits and vegetables: superheroes!

Fresh fruit and vegetables, even lightly steamed or roasted vegetables, are an indispensable part of your weight loss and overall health plan. I realized I needed to take seriously the CDC's recommendation to eat four to six servings of fruits and vegetables *daily*. Not only are the fruits and vegetables filling and unbeatable for snacks, they also are loaded with nutrients, fiber, some protein, and antioxidants. These antioxidants reduce the inflammation that causes belly fat and a host of other conditions. According to a recent study out of the Linus Pauling Institute at Oregon State University,[xxv] cruciferous vegetables offer many cancer-fighting benefits. The National Cancer Institute also advises us to include these cancer fighters in our quest for good health.

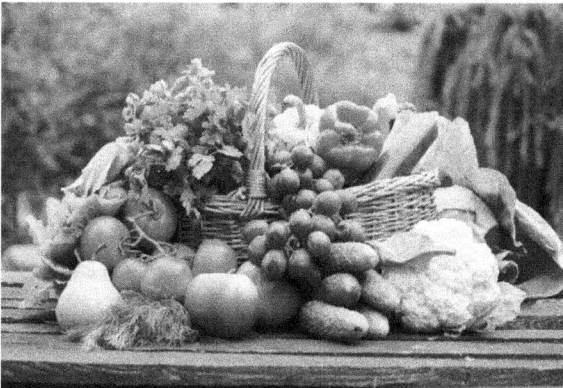

As a result of these proven health perks, we have been eating far more of these fat/cancer/inflammation fighters over the past couple of years. You should, too. The cool cruciferous crew of which I speak are broccoli, cauliflower, kale, red cabbage, mustard and collard greens, turnips and turnip greens, arugula, and watercress - yes, I know, I reached back to the '60s for that one. Also, give Brussels sprouts another chance. They are delicious if you roast them. Don't forget the other colors of the veggie rainbow—the red, yellow, and orange bell peppers, red tomatoes, beets, radicchio, onions, radishes, orange carrots, sweet potatoes, and of course, butternut and yellow squash.

Select from this list for your lunch and dinner veggies, and you can't go wrong. Again, overcooked veggies are a waste. Don't get me wrong, I know most of you are not going to eat the Brussels sprouts raw. That reality is in no way lost on me. Just lightly steam or roast them (toss the sprouts or your favorite veggies onto a cookie sheet, drizzle a tad bit of salt and olive oil on top, along with your favorite herbs, and slide them into the oven at 350 degrees for about ten to thirty minutes, depending on the vegetable). You can always run cool water over the frozen vegetables to thaw them, then sauté the veggies in a small amount of water over medium heat for a couple of minutes. If you do boil them, bring them to a boil, and then simmer just for a few minutes. Yes, those veggies should still be crunchy, not mushy. If they're mushy and your pot water or "pot liquor" is the color of the vegetables cooked, then your punishment is to drink the green, orange or purple water. By doing so, you are drinking the nutrients that boiled into the water.

Note: Although nearly all of our fruits and veggies are organic, we wash them as thoroughly as we washed their nonorganic counterparts.

TWO MINUTE DRILL!

CHAPTER 6

Meal Planning

**Which of you desiring to build a tower does not
first sit down to count the cost?**
LUKE 14:28

S
uccessful weight loss involves three basic concepts: (1) eliminating the
foods and obesogens that are keeping us fat; (2) eating the right foods
for your meals and snacks; and (3) incorporating enough movement and
activity in your life to trigger the muscle contraction that regulates insulin, revs
metabolism, and burns fat. I must admit that changing one's diet and lifestyle
is not as easy as it sounds. Over the course of the year, I discovered that nearly
forty percent of my meals and snacks were eaten outside of the home. Many of
us eat outside of the home for two to three meals and snacks each day. On the
weekends, we get together for birthday parties, anniversaries, weddings, sporting
events, movies, and of course, dinners and brunches. The secret to my success
was managing what I do both inside and outside of the home. That management
process starts here.

PLAN YOUR MEALS...AND YOUR SNACKS!
Recapturing, or discovering for the first time, the glory days requires planning.
Plan five to seven different breakfasts, lunches, and dinners. Equally as important
as the meals, identify the top five to seven snacks that work for you. This planning takes time. Are you catching on? I suggest reserving one "two-day" each

month for two or three months to really get your program off the ground. Please tell me you are willing to carve out this time for your health and vitality.

Budget your macros (protein, fiber, fat, carbohydrates) and sugar.

As you plan your meals and snacks, tally the healthy fats, fiber, protein and sugar grams provided by the day's meals and snacks. We plan how to spend our money (at least we're supposed to). Apply that principle to our nutritional limits. For example, just as I have only ten dollars or twenty dollars to spend today without overdrawing my account (resulting in thirty-nine dollars in bounced-check fees), I can spend only 100–120 carbohydrate grams, or twenty-five to thirty sugar grams. Likewise, if you know you need around fifty protein grams per day, plan your meals and snacks to ensure they contain your daily requirement of protein. In fact, your plan needs to add up to your daily limits of all of your macronutrients. Then shop for the ingredients.

On average, I ate around one-quarter of my protein (twelve to fifteen grams), fat (twelve to fifteen grams), carbohydrates (twenty to twenty-five grams), and fiber (five to six grams) in my breakfast foods. Initially, I needed to count these macronutrients to make sure I budgeted correctly. Eventually, I began to do the math in my head. Imagine that!

Lose the retro meals!

As I started this transformative lifestyle change, I realized that I am a product of both my upbringing and the traditional notions of what constitutes a well-balanced meal. To lose the weight, I needed to revise my notion of what constitutes breakfast, lunch, snacks, and dinner. I had to *loosen the grip that tradition had on my typical diet.* For example, when we think of the traditional dinner plate, it often contained meatloaf, fried chicken, or pork chops, mashed potatoes, and a vegetable (usually overcooked), along with a slice of bread and butter. That was the past. Now, my reconstituted dinner plate often contains:

(1) Grilled fish (wild-caught salmon, cod, flounder) *instead of fried anything*
(2) Starchy vegetable such as carrots, cauliflower, sweet potato, or a *small* serving of a whole grain such as brown rice, quinoa, or other 100 percent whole-grain pasta *instead of white rice, white potato, and most pasta* (sorry, part of my weight-loss journey involved ditching all egg noodles)

(3) *Two* servings of vegetables, including a leafy green veggie such as Brussels sprouts, kale, collard greens, mustard greens, or lightly sautéed spinach *and* sliced tomatoes, cucumbers, and onion, broccoli, or a salad.

In addition, I realized I was most successful when I identified the foods I ate regularly and determined what nutritional value those foods contributed. A useful tracking tool can be found at https://www.supertracker.usda.gov. This website provides the nutritional content for many of the foods we consume daily.

Organic fruits and veggies: the new bread!
Didn't she just write a dissertation on fruits and vegetables in Chapter 5? Consider this the encore. Organic fruits and vegetables are on the front line of the *JustForMeDiet* plan. This is because recent studies suggest that organic fruits and veggies have from 18–69 percent ***more antioxidants*** (thus deserving an underline, bold, and italics!) than the pesticide versions of our produce.[xxvi] More antioxidants mean less inflammation. Lower your inflammation and you shrink your belly. Hello!

How many apples a day did you say?
We all know we're supposed to eat four to six servings (or cups) of fruits and vegetables per day. The CDC defines one cup as follows: *one apple, one bell pepper, eight medium strawberries, one small wedge of watermelon, a large orange, two or three plums, two medium carrots, one large sweet potato, one cup cooked greens, or two cups raw greens.*[xxvii] By the way, I know we have been told that we can substitute a glass of orange juice or apple juice as one serving of fruit, but not in the *JustForMeDiet*. Sorry.

****

JUSTFORME TIP: *I Cannot Eat Greens Because I Take Blood Thinners.*
If you are taking blood thinners and your vitamin K intake is restricted, consult your doctor before adding any greens to your smoothie or to your diet. These no-no's include spinach, parsley, broccoli, kale, cilantro, avocado, and even non-green blueberries. Ask your doctor about chopped cauliflower and carrots for great nutrition instead of greens. To supplement the missing fiber, consider black beans, chia seeds, oranges, nectarines, lima beans, apricots, cherries, pineapples, and shitake mushrooms. Always be sure to consult with your doctor before making dietary changes.

****

MEAL PLANS

BREAKFAST

As early as I can remember, I was taught that breakfast is the most important meal of the day. Breakfast will set the tone for the day—for good or for bad. Needless to say, that tone depends on what you eat and drink or don't eat and drink for breakfast. From personal experience, I learned that two doughnuts or a high-sodium, high-carb, high-trans-fat breakfast biscuit started my day on a path to weight gain and brain fog, while a healthy veggie omelet or a bowl of oatmeal with fruit and nuts started my day with energy, mental clarity, and a long-lasting feeling of fullness. What you eat for breakfast is as important as having breakfast.

Breakfast of champions?

The typical American breakfast plate consists of sugary yogurt, high-carb cereal, or low-protein, low-fiber bread products such as doughnuts, toast, pancakes, or waffles (usually processed), or even fast food or microwavable breakfast sandwiches and orange juice. On the weekends, breakfast consists of eggs/bacon or sausage (whether pork, turkey, or even soy), biscuits, or toast (French or American), fried potatoes, or grits smothered in margarine—you know, partially hydrogenated vegetable oil. Trans fat, carbohydrates, and sugar all comprise the common denominator.

I finally learned that weight loss success involved designing meal and snack plans that incorporated the recommended amounts of fruits and vegetables, protein, fiber and healthy fats. I also realized it all starts with breakfast. I usually manage to eat at least one to two servings of fruit or veggies by noon—whether in the form of an apple in my oatmeal, one to two servings of veggies and herbs added to my scrambled eggs, or guacamole and organic tortilla chips for a noon snack. At breakfast, instead of toast, I have a serving of fruit. Instead of bread with dinner, I add the additional vegetable.

As I started the *JustForMeDiet*, I realized I needed to eliminate the multiple servings of heavy carbs and ensure that I incorporated twelve to fifteen grams of protein, on average, and around twelve to fifteen grams of healthy fat with each meal. I started by substituting the high-carb/low-fiber cereals, breads, potatoes, or grits with one to two servings of fruit and veggies for breakfast. I also incorporated organic plain nonfat Greek or regular plain nonfat yogurt. I still had to watch the sugars, however, because even one eight-ounce container of organic *flavored* Greek yogurt contained anywhere from twelve to twenty grams of sugar.

****
JUSTFORME TIP: I'm Allergic to Dairy Products
Many people who are allergic to milk products can still eat yogurt, and there are lactose-free yogurts on the market. But if you cannot eat yogurt from cow's milk, try coconut yogurt. It is tasty and healthy.
****

These are some of the meals that worked for me:

THE *JUSTFORME* BREAKFAST MENU

- Oatmeal + fourteen walnut halves + one medium chopped apple + one teaspoon cinnamon + two ounces of almond milk + one-half cup berries (again, I prefer organic, and thawed frozen berries are fine), *instead of 1.5 bowls of "healthy" but heavily carbed cold cereal and sugary milk* (even fat-free organic milk contains twelve grams of sugar per cup.)

- Plain Greek yogurt + blueberries + walnuts + one teaspoon coconut sugar or one packet organic stevia (for those who like it sweet, like me); coffee or tea

- One or two scrambled eggs (preferably organic)+ leftover salmon (fish for breakfast is a staple in the Caribbean and other parts of the world) + a handful of grapes (didn't you know? Grapes or berries are the new toast]) + coffee (with an ounce of almond milk)

- One apple with two tablespoons peanut butter or almond butter + coffee

- One slice of high-fiber (four to six grams per slice), high-protein (four to six grams per slice) organic bread + two tbsp. peanut butter

- Smoothie (with or without greens)—almond or organic milk + six ounces of organic plain Greek or regular nonfat yogurt + one-quarter cup fresh berries + seven to eight walnuts, a handful of flax or other seeds, almonds, or two tablespoons peanut butter. This is *your* smoothie! Experiment with what makes you happy. From bananas and spinach to mangos, wheat germ and chia seeds—you control the smoothie. Again, if **it is replacing a meal, be sure** to cover the bases in protein, fiber, and healthy fat.

- One to two boiled eggs with raspberries + 1 turkey sausage link

- One banana with 2 tbsp. peanut butter + 2 turkey sausage links

Note: Organic berries are not cheap. However, you can find them frozen in bulk at the bulk discount stores. Call the bulk chains in your region and ask if they are in stock. If not, ask them to start carrying the berries or at least tell you which stores carry them. The frozen organic berries at these stores might be cheaper than the nonorganic brands at regular grocery stores.

Cold breakfast cereals—a changing of the guard

Most of you reading this book probably will not stop buying cold breakfast cereal. You have children, or you simply do not have the time each morning to prepare a healthier breakfast. Here are some options. Again, the aim is a healthy carbohydrate-protein-fiber ratio, along with a low sugar content. I listed some of the cold cereals that have good macronutrient ratios and that also are reasonably low in sugar. This list is by no means exhaustive. There are other great selections on the grocery shelves, particularly in the organic aisle.

1 serving cereal	Carbs	Fiber	Protein	Sugars
Fiber One (original)	25	14	2	0
Kashi's GOLEAN	40	13	12	8
Nature's Path Optimum Slim	40	9	9	6
Cascadian Farms Hearty Morning	38	8	4	8
Shredded Wheat	37	6	5	0
Wheat Chex	39	6	5	5
Wheaties	22	3	2	4
Cheerios	20	3	3	1

Again, protein is king and fiber is queen (I suppose healthy fat is prince?) because they zap my appetite for the entire morning and even for the first part of the afternoon. When I finally do eat lunch, I'm really not that hungry.

LUNCH

In all likelihood, you eat lunch outside of your home. Most of you left home early this morning to get to work or to get kids to school, and the plan for lunch involved going out to eat, right? That's about to change, and it is not difficult. Also get ready to save some money! Like many of you, I ate out for lunch most days of the week. Because lunch constitutes 33 percent of our meals and is the only meal eaten outside of the home nearly 100 percent of the time, it requires discussion and planning. In a nutshell, just as you plan your wardrobe from the clothing to the accessories, take the time to plan the 33 percent otherwise known as "lunch."

Lose the lunch crowd...Lose the weight!
My work friends are not going to be happy with this section! I have observed that one of the biggest saboteurs to weight loss is the lunch crowd. Yes, our colleagues or work buddies go out to lunch nearly every day. Joining them, however, will require you to tap your calorie, carb, fat, and sugar "budget" reserves several times per week. Let's be clear: this crowd does not gain weight. They usually are in the gym after work for a solid hour or more, and do not have to drive an hour or longer during rush hour traffic to arrive at their kids' baseball games or dance rehearsals. And they probably are not going to cook dinner after sitting at the two-hour game.

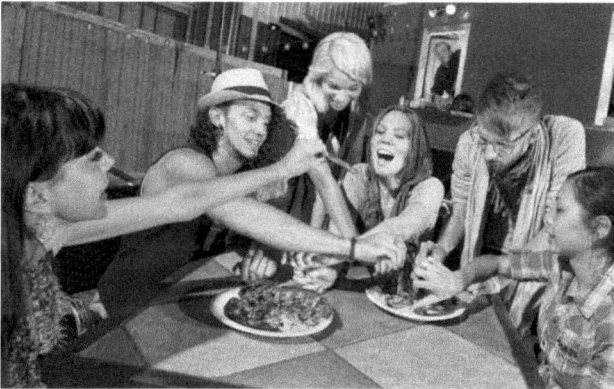

Here's the point: the lunch crowd has some luxuries most of us don't have: time, money, and supercharged metabolisms to burn off all of those fries and strawberry lemonades. So, forgetaboutit! Again, you need to control every meal. We claim we don't have the money to purchase organic or other healthier foods. Actually, we do, but we burn the money while hanging with the lunch crowd. The lunch crowd will not be happy you are cutting the ties. But you must. For the tens of millions of us who have primarily a sedentary job, our half- or full- hour lunchtime is a key break during which we can stop the sedentary stupor and walk three thousand to four thousand of the ten thousand steps we should take per day. Now that you have parted company with the lunch crowd (or invited them to join you for your lunch walks), let's have lunch:

JUSTFORME LUNCH MENU

Since most of us are in the workforce, running with kids, or otherwise starved of the time needed to make healthy lunches, here are examples of quick lunches that contain the healthy trinity—protein, fiber, and healthy fat:

- Tuna salad + an apple (once every couple of weeks because of the risk of mercury found in tuna)
- Homemade salad + leftover salmon or lean chicken or turkey lunch meat (with no nitrates or nitrites) + vinaigrette dressing
- Chili over one-quarter cup brown rice or served with about seven to eight organic tortilla chips + vegetable salad + vinaigrette dressing
- Chicken soup + organic whole grain crackers or organic tortilla chips + sliced avocado + an apple
- Peanut butter on pita chips + a cucumber and red onion salad + two tablespoons of vinaigrette dressing
- One-half cup organic refried beans (once in a while) + one-half cup guacamole + organic tortilla chips (no more than ten) with an apple
- Plain Greek yogurt (low fat) + walnuts or almonds + fruit added
- A turkey, egg salad, or tuna sandwich on one slice of organic high- fiber/high-protein bread + cucumber slices, lettuce, basil, broccoli sprouts (one to one-half servings of veggies if possible) + one tablespoon soy-free mayo or mustard, or half an avocado as the sandwich spread + an apple
- Dinner leftovers!

Note: During the first four months of my diet, I rarely ate two slices of bread at one sitting. When I did, the bread was one hundred percent whole grain and contained at least three grams of fiber per slice.

DINNER

Similar to lunch, dinner in the United States has transformed over the past couple of decades. Remember the days when the whole family sat down together at the dinner table? We talked about work, school, upcoming events, politics, church, and football (of course!). According to some studies, the "talking" part of the meal actually slowed digestion because we would eat food, chew, and then talk in between bites. Slowing digestion allows your body to realize it is full, so we would actually eat less and minimize carb overload, insulin resistance, and sugar spikes, thereby helping to keep us slimmer. Who knew! These days, dinner is on the fly; it consists of fast food or it is ordered in. Rarely do we sit down as a family, and our waists have paid the price. Enough sermonizing. Below are meals that did their part in peeling the weight off of my hips:

JUSTFORME DINNER MENU

- Grilled salmon (four ounces wild caught or sockeye) + roasted Brussels sprouts + sweet potatoes with cinnamon, nutmeg, extra virgin olive or coconut oil, and one teaspoon of organic coconut sugar if you need the sweetness (instead of margarine and brown sugar)
- Baked cod or haddock (four ounces) with lemon juice, vinaigrette marinade + black beans + broccoli mixed with cauliflower
- Organic baked chicken (four ounces) + salad with organic low-sugar or soy-free vinaigrette dressing + cauliflower mashed with salt, pepper, and olive oil or a tad bit of organic butter
- Chili with ground turkey, black or kidney bean chili (we add garlic, red onions, rosemary, oregano, turmeric, salt, pepper, and chili powder) + quinoa + garden salad + two tablespoons vinaigrette dressing + collard greens with apple cider vinegar and crushed red peppers
- Shrimp stir fry cooked in one tablespoon coconut oil with fresh ginger + brown rice + lots of tasty organic stir-fried vegetables cooked in herbs
- Organic roast chicken + red or green cabbage + brown rice or sautéed yams
- Oatmeal—just checking to see if you were paying attention. (Actually, oatmeal for dinner once in a while will work wonders on the scale.)
- Spaghetti + one small serving of quinoa, brown rice or 100 percent whole-grain noodles + organic tomato basil sauce (store bought or homemade) containing organic ground turkey meat

FOR RED MEAT EATERS
Again, my physician advised that I reduce or eliminate altogether my red meat intake because of the animal fat. As a result, red meat dinner suggestions are limited in the *JustForMeDiet* plan.

- Lean steak (from grass-fed cows and with no hormones or antibiotics) + one-half cup organic succotash + one of cup kale
- Lamb chops (my weakness!)+ salad + spinach + quinoa
- Meat loaf + roasted carrots and bell peppers + garden salad with vinaigrette dressing

SNACKS

We cannot discuss meals without a few words about snacks. For many of us, the war on weight is lost at snack time. Snacks are an important part of the American diet. Many of us eat lunch at noon. By 3:00 p.m., we crash. Most of us don't leave work until 5:30 p.m. or 6:00 p.m. or later. After the hour-long commute, it's 7:00 p.m. or 8:00 p.m. by the time we get home. Then, unless you pop a frozen dish into the microwave for dinner (*that's a whole 'nother issue*), another thirty to forty-five minutes passes before you sit down to eat. In the past, I was famished by the time I crossed the threshold at home and would eat the first thing I could find. Okay, I would carb out! When I began to bring healthy, sustaining snacks (filled with a decent dose of fiber and/or protein) to work to eat during the mid-afternoon slump or toward the end of the workday, I eliminated the "carb crashes" and was able to wait until dinner was served before eating again.

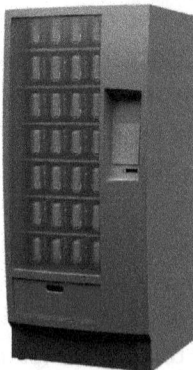

Avoid land mines.

The mid-morning and mid-afternoon crashes, even the nighttime snack attack, are land mines. If you *plan in advance* to eat four to five times per day, you will be prepared. If you do not plan ahead and stock up on the *JustForMeDiet* healthy snacks in your pantry, your car, at your desk, or in your book bag or purse, you will step into a land mine...the vending machine, the candy jar in the office, or the office kitchen with the leftover pizza or doughnuts from the staff meeting. There is nothing, I repeat, *nothing* in the vending machine (not even the BPA-laced water bottle!) worth selecting that will help you lose weight. Don't do it!

****
JUSTFORME TIP: *Someone Else Does My Grocery Shopping*
This scenario presents an opportunity for you to educate the shopper about making healthier food selections. Ask to accompany the shopper to the grocery store, and point out the differences between the healthy and not-so-healthy products so the shopper will make the right choice.
****

Snacks I select!
I have created a repertoire of snacks that contain a decent amount of protein and/or fiber while low on carbs and sugar. I buy them in bulk to keep with me for those long afternoon stretches in between meals. Here are my favorites. You can choose from this list or create your own list that has factored your nutritional budget.

JUSTFORME SNACK MENU

- Apples (feel free to spoon some peanut butter on them) and oranges
- Berries
- Bananas with peanut butter
- Mini or chopped veggies
- Homemade trail mix
- Lite organic popcorn
- Guacamole and organic tortilla chips (one half cup will fill you up). Grocery stores now sell prepackaged organic guacamole. You can always make your own.
- Yogurt
- A handful of nuts
- Kale chips (make your own!)
- Organic snack bars (low-sugar, high-fiber)

Below are some of the snack bars that fit the fiber and protein bill for me.

Organic or Non-GMO bars

Let's face it, we all occasionally need some sort of snack bar, granola bar, or protein bar (I refuse to say candy bar) to get through the day. I have searched high and low and found some soy-free, or at least the organic soy brands. You can also check out www.lifesoyfree.com for more suggestions. Here are some of my go-to bars:

➢ Cascadian Farms Organic Peanut Butter Chocolate Chip protein granola bars (9 g of protein, 3 g fiber, 11 g sugar) per www.cascadiafarms.com
➢ Clif Bar—Kit's Organic Dark Chocolate Almond Coconut (4 g protein, 5 g fiber, 15 g sugar) per www.clifbar.com
➢ Clif Bar—Kit's Organic Dark Chocolate Peanut (5 g protein, 4 g fiber, 18 g sugar) per www.clifbar.com
➢ Nature's Path Organic Coconut Chia Granola (5 g protein, 6 g fiber, 9 g sugar) www.naturespath.com
➢ NuGo Free Dark Chocolate Crunch Bars (9 g protein, 4 g fiber, 11 g sugar) per www.nugo.com

These brands have various other delicious flavors. As you can see, I lean toward chocolate, almonds, and coconut...

Note: Always remember to read the ingredient list to ensure the products do not contain your particular allergen, such as nuts or dairy.

****

JUSTFORME TIP: I Have Fibroid Tumors

Many women have fibroid tumors or ovarian cysts. I try to limit my soy intake because soy mimics estrogen in the body, and it is believed to contribute to the growth of fibroid tumors.

****

A WEEK IN THE LIFE OF THE JUSTFORMEDIET

In addition to the list of meals I provided earlier, I wanted you to see how these meals come together to meet my macronutrient needs throughout the day.

These macronutrient and sugar-gram contents (rounded to the nearest half gram) reflect estimates that are based on package labels and product website nutritional guides, which often differ from brand to brand for the same food item. For example, some egg companies record six grams of protein per egg while other brands record seven grams. Therefore, these estimates might vary slightly from the brands you use. A complete chart of the macronutrient content of the foods provided in this meal plan can be found in Appendix B.

The *JustForMeDiet* One-Week Meal Plan

<u>SUNDAY</u>
BREAKFAST: 23 g protein, 7 g fiber, 23 g fat, 23 g carbs, 13.5 g sugar

- 6 oz. organic plain nonfat Greek yogurt
- Walnuts, blueberries, and stevia
- Coffee with milk and stevia

SNACK: 3 g protein, 6.5 g fiber, 23 g fat, 27 g carbs

- 1/2 cup guacamole
- 1 small serving of organic tortilla chips
- Tall glass of lazy-girl lemonade

DINNER: 33 g protein, 9.5 g fiber, 8.5 g fat, 36 g carbs, 7 g sugar

- 1/2 skinless roast chicken breast
- 1 medium sweet potato with 1 tbsp. Smart Balance Buttery Spread (olive oil), cinnamon, and nutmeg
- 1 cup of lightly steamed broccoli
- Cooled berry tea with stevia and mint leaves added

DESSERT: 1 g protein, 3 g fiber, 2 g fat, 17 g carbs, 7 g sugar

- Cascadia Farms Organic Oatmeal Raisin Granola Bar

DAILY TOTAL: 60 g protein, 26 g fiber, 56.5 g fat, 103 g carbs, 27.5 g sugar

MONDAY

BREAKFAST: 11.5 g protein, 10 g fiber, 19 g fat, 59 g carbs, 12 g sugar

- 1 serving of cooked oatmeal with stevia
- 1/2 apple, 1 tbsp. cinnamon
- 1/4 cup almonds
- 2 oz. low-fat organic milk and green tea

LUNCH: 22 g protein, 6 g fiber, 5.5 g fat, 24 g carbs, 4.5 g sugar

- Sunday's dinner leftovers (2/3 serving)

SNACK: 2 g fiber, 12.5 g carbs, 9.5 g sugar

- Rest of the apple

DINNER: 30 g protein, 4.5 g fiber, 15 g fat, 29.5 g carbs, 6 g sugar

- 4 oz. filet grilled salmon
- 1 cup salad with romaine lettuce and/or kale, cucumbers, red onions, red bell peppers with 2 tbsp. balsamic vinaigrette
- 1/2 cup of quinoa

DAILY TOTAL: *63.5 g protein, 22.5 g fiber, 39.5 g fat, 125 carbs, 32 g sugar*

TUESDAY

BREAKFAST: 15.5 g protein, 10.5 g fiber, 21.5 g fat, 45 g carbs, 12 g sugar

- 1 serving of cooked oatmeal with stevia
- 1/2 apple, 1 tbsp. cinnamon
- 1/2 oz. almonds (around 11 or 12 almonds)
- 2 oz. low-fat organic milk and green tea

LUNCH: 28 g protein, 4 g fiber, 21 g fat, 25 g carbs, 5.5 g sugar

- Tuna salad and crackers

DINNER: 20 g protein, 11.5 g fiber, 12 g fat, 26.5 g carbs, 2.5 g sugar

- 3 oz. American lamb (leg steak)
- 1 cup cooked spinach, sautéed in spray EVOO with 2 oz. water, red onions, crushed red pepper, and garlic
- 1 cup steamed cauliflower
- 1 tall glass of lazy-girl limeade with two packets of stevia and fresh lime juice

DAILY TOTAL: 63.5 g protein, 26 g fiber, 54.5 g fat, 96.5 g carbs, 20 g sugar

WEDNESDAY

BREAKFAST: 13 g protein, 10.5 g fiber, 17 g fat, 23 g carbs, 3 g sugar

- 1 slice organic high-fiber/high-protein (soy-free) bread
- 2 tbsp. peanut butter
- Coffee or tea with two packets of stevia

LUNCH: 28 g protein, 4 g fiber, 21 g fat, 25 g carbs, 5.5 g sugar

- 3 oz. tuna salad with 1/2 cup diced red onions and apples, cilantro with 1 tbsp. organic mayo
- 10 Mary's Gone Black Pepper crackers

DINNER: 22.5 g protein, 11 g fiber, 5.5 g fat, 58 carbs, 5.5 g sugar

- 1 cup turkey chili with black beans
- 1/2 cup brown rice and 1 tbsp non-GMO Smart Balance buttery spread with extra virgin olive oil (EVOO)
- 1.5 cup lettuce/vegetable salad with 2 tbsp. balsamic vinaigrette

DAILY TOTAL: 63.5 g protein, 25.5 g fiber, 43.5 g fat, 106 g carbs, 14 g sugar

THURSDAY

BREAKFAST: 15 g protein, 3.5 g fiber, 15 g fat, 18 g carbs, 13 g sugar

- 2 scrambled eggs cooked in spray EVOO with 1 cup spinach

- 1/2 cup of grapes
- Hot herbal tea sweetened with stevia, if necessary

LUNCH: 22.5 g protein, 11 g fiber, 5.5 g fat, 58 g carbs, 5.5 g sugar

- Wednesday's dinner leftovers

DINNER: 24 g protein, 9.5 g fiber, 5 g fat, 49 g carbs, 7.5 g sugar

- Southwest Chicken Salad: 1 quarter boneless, skinless grilled chicken breast, cubed
- 1/2 cup black beans
- 1/2 cup organic whole kernel corn
- 2 tbsp. vinaigrette dressing
- 5 organic tortilla chips, crumbled

DAILY TOTAL: *61.5 g protein, 24 g fiber, 25.5 g fat, 125 g carbs, 26 g sugar*

FRIDAY

BREAKFAST: 23 g protein, 7 g fiber, 23 g fat, 23 g carbs, 12.5 g sugar

- 6 oz. organic plain nonfat Greek yogurt
- Walnuts, blueberries, and two packets of stevia
- Coffee with milk and stevia

LUNCH: 23.5 g protein, 15 g fiber, 9 g fat, 44.5 g carbs, 8.5 g sugar

- Turkey sandwich with 1 serving sliced turkey breast, 1 slice Swiss cheese, 6–7 basil leaves, black pepper on
- 2 slices double-fiber bread
- 2 tbsp. guacamole as the sandwich spread
- 1/2 cup assorted raw veggies such as sliced bell peppers, grape tomatoes, broccoli, and carrots
- Balsamic vinaigrette (*you didn't think I ate the veggies plain, did you?*)

SNACK: 1 g protein, 2 g fiber, .5 g fat, 10.5 g carbs, 7.5 g sugar

- 1 cup blueberries (bring them to work in a small sealable container)

DINNER: 32 g protein, 9 g fiber, 18 g fat, 28 g carbs, 2 g sugar

- 4 oz. grilled whiting
- 1/2 cup cauliflower mash cooked with organic nonfat buttermilk, garlic, light salt/pepper
- 1 cup kale
- Water with lemon and/or lime

DAILY TOTAL: *79.5 g protein, 33 g fiber, 50.5 g fat, 106 g carbs, 30.5 g sugar*

SATURDAY
BRUNCH: 26.5 g protein, 15 g fiber, 22.5 g fat, 42.5 g carbs, 14.5 g sugar

- 2 scrambled eggs cooked in EVOO spray and FILLED with veggies and herbs including basil, rosemary, onions, bell peppers, and broccoli
- 2 organic turkey sausage patties
- 1 slice high-fiber toast with strawberry compote (1/4 cup strawberries sautéed in a few tbsp. water with 2 packets of stevia)
- 1/2 cup of grapes
- Coffee with 2 oz. organic low-fat milk and stevia

MIDAFTERNOON SNACK: 3 g protein, 5 g fiber, 4 g fat, 17 g carbs, 1 g sugar

- 1 cup organic coconut popcorn

DINNER: 30 g protein, 8 g fiber, 20 g fat, 20 g carbs, 6 g sugar

- Sautéed shrimp with 1 scallion
- 1/2 cup green peas, ginger, turmeric, sautéed with shrimp in 1 tbsp. EVOO spray
- 1 cup salad with raw vegetables with 2 tbsp. balsamic vinaigrette

DESSERT: 4 g protein, 5 g fiber, 12 g fat, 26 g carbs, 15 g sugar

- Kit's Organic Dark Chocolate Almond Coconut Bar

DAILY TOTAL: *63.5 g protein, 33 g fiber, 58.5 g fat, 105.5 carbs, 36.5 g sugar*

Now, it's your turn to create tasty and filling meals and snacks from the *JustForMeDiet* foods using the WEEK IN THE LIFE worksheet found at www. Thejustformediet.com.

****

JUSTFORME TIP: I Don't Have a Refrigerator at Work.
Thank GOD for thermoses and insulated lunch bags. They do a much better job than plastic or paper bags at keeping your food cold. You can also insert frozen pack gels into your lunch container to minimize the risk of food-borne illnesses.

****

CHAPTER 7

We Need Bodyguards!

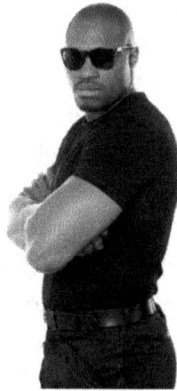

No weapon that is formed against me shall prosper.
ISAIAH 54:17

Hip-hop moguls aren't the only ones who need bodyguards. I avoid eating any processed carbs, bad fat, or sugar items without first reaching for protection from *my bodyguard!* Huh? Isn't that a movie? In fact, there are foods and substances that you can eat or drink before our main meal that serve as "damage control" by slowing digestion to give your body the time it needs to absorb the sugar or glucose, particularly if you are about to indulge in something not found in this book (I'll leave it at that).[xxviii] Below is a list of the foods I have found to be filling, tasty, filled with fiber, protein, or healthy fats and, thus, will slow digestion and minimize the damage to our health.

❖ **MY BODYGUARDS:**

1. **Apple cider vinegar:** one tablespoon with one glass of water twenty minutes before your meals or before heading out to the food fest.
2. **Fresh vegetables:** keep a big bowl of cut broccoli, cauliflower, bell peppers, celery, cucumbers and carrots in the fridge and baggie some up on your way out the door—eat them in the car before you walk into the "dessert-only" reception (dessert only? Can you say, diabetic shock?).
3. **Avocado or guacamole:** I'll spread guacamole on five to six organic tortilla chips before I leave home.
4. **Fresh or frozen berries:** organic, please! They are loaded in antioxidants.
5. **Black /kidney beans**: my cabinet is stocked with BPA-free pop top cans of black beans—I literally will grab one on the go, pop it open, and eat right out of the can—please don't tell my mother! Stock up on these and other legumes.
6. **Peanut or almond butter:** I used to come home and "carb" out, but now I come home and have one tablespoon of peanut butter or almond butter. It calms the savage beast, for real, for real!
7. **Apples:** they are loaded with fiber. I take one to work with me nearly every day, and I reach for it when I get hungry—you know, at 3:00 p.m. or even from 5:00–6:00 p.m., as the workday draws to a close. Those apples, along with the thought of the sugar, excess carbs, chemicals and preservatives, keep me out of the vending machines.
8. **Oatmeal:** learn to love this heavenly food—I kid you not, I'll eat some oatmeal before going to a cookout or a birthday bash where I know diet saboteurs are lying in wait for me.
9. **Nuts and seeds:** good for you, but just don't overdo it.
10. **Green tea:** remember, it contains caffeine.
11. **Lemon and lime juice, and zest:** if you zest, please wash the fruit first.
12. **Salad with vinaigrette or Italian dressing:** please measure your serving of dressing, syrup, sauce, and jelly. Also, from this day forward, use *only* vinaigrette or Italian dressing (or oil and vinegar) until the weight is gone.
13. **Cinnamon and turmeric:** they lower blood sugar and offer other amazing health properties. Cinnamon tells the brain it's getting something sweet.

14. **Organic plain Greek yogurt:** yes, I said "plain" and I didn't stutter. If the organic brands are not available, I buy yogurt derived from grass-fed cows with no added hormones or antibiotics.
15. **Water:** drink a couple of glasses of water before eating and you will be too full to overindulge!

Note: I prefer to add the turmeric spice to my food instead of taking the supplement. Turmeric is a strong anti-inflammatory and has blood-thinning properties.

****

JUSTFORME TIP: I Have Acid Reflux, and Lemon Juice Upsets My Stomach.
  I suffered with a brief bout of acid reflux a couple of years ago. I found that an ounce of apple cider vinegar mixed with four ounces of water soothed my bouts of acid reflux. Ginger tea and extract in water also helped my stomach heal from acid reflux.
****

I put this bodyguard list to the test. I went on vacation to a Caribbean resort and I ate to my heart's content. Before every meal, however, I ate a handful of walnuts, drank lemon or lime water, and at dinner ate a salad with vinaigrette dressing before the main course. After eight days, I did not gain weight. I know what you're thinking: "You didn't lose weight either." Well, you try *losing* weight while vacationing at a Caribbean resort for eight days!

Stock up

Why is stocking up on your bodyguards important? If these bodyguards are in your house, you will begin to eat them. You will have them on hand to take with you when you leave for work, church, or wherever you go. These are the food items that will keep you full, slow sugar spikes, and give you maximum protein/fiber/healthy fats and other vital nutrients. These are the foods, condiments, sweeteners, or flavorings that will replace the unhealthy condiments, sugars, and snacks that have made us what we were - overweight and unhealthy. If they are not readily accessible, we tend to reach for whatever is close by—whether it is a candy bar or chips in the vending machine or the doughnuts in the office kitchen.

❖ DAMAGE CONTROL: MORE WAYS TO INCREASE FAT BURNING AND REVERSE WEIGHT GAIN

Drink more water

In order to lose the weight, keep it off, and obtain maximum health, you need to learn to drink water. There is really no way around this requirement. I wish I could tell you that water is not an essential part of this process, but I would be lying to you. I drink eight to ten glasses of water (notice I said glasses, not water bottles). Water's benefits are discussed in chapter 9, called "Lose the Liquid Pounds." One benefit worth mentioning here is that water helps to reduce body fat.

Avoid carb overload!

Avoid eating too many carbs in the same meal, even if you don't exceed your daily limit. It looks something like this: We go out to a breakfast buffet. In addition to the bacon and scrambled eggs, we order biscuits, butter, and jelly (or pancakes with butter or margarine with a gallon of syrup), grits *and/or* fried potatoes, orange juice ("Large, please"), and a few packs of sugar in our coffee with high-fat creamer. Hmmm, how about 150 grams of carbohydrates, fifty-plus grams of fat, and about ninety grams of sugar, which is over three times the sugar limit for the average person as recommended by the American Heart Association.

Mama Mia!

Or, we go to the local Italian restaurant and order the strawberry lemonade (sixty-five to seventy grams of sugar and about seventy grams of carbs in the tall glass—that's before the free refill), two to three breadsticks (about ninety carb grams!), the Caesar salad with the three hundred-calorie dressing already on the salad, and the main course—the fettuccine Alfredo (nearly one hundred carb grams, filled with nearly fifty saturated fat grams! Don't forget the nearly fourteen hundred sodium grams—what I like to call...*insta-stroke!*). Oops, I forgot about dessert (one serving of tiramisu has about thirty sugar grams and forty carb grams)...Get the point? Do the math—this meal delivered a whopping three hundred carbohydrate grams (roughly) and around *ninety* sugar grams... before we even talk about saturated fat and sodium.

The result? More than twice your carb limit for the day...in one meal, otherwise known as "carb overload." Even without the sugar, you experience a sugar spike, insulin resistance, and a setback to your weight-loss program. On the other hand, as you begin to dial down the carbs, the sugars, the unhealthy fats, and begin to make the healthy trinity a regular part of your diet, the weight *will* come off, and your risk of suffering from these unhealthy conditions will diminish.

Lower your glycemic load.

I learned to lower my glycemic load—the amount of carbohydrates in the food in relation to their impact on blood sugar levels. We now know that a high refined carb intake is the culprit that typically causes a spike in blood sugar or glucose, an outcome worsened by our sedentary lifestyles. Foods with a low glycemic index usually contain fiber, protein, or healthy fat (the healthy trinity). These foods will slow the metabolism of carbohydrates, and minimize insulin resistance, and they have been shown to help control type 2 diabetes and improve weight loss. The name of the game is to fill your grocery cart with low glycemic foods.

Beans, lentils, nuts, fruit, vegetables, whole grains, fish, and lean meats generally are lower on the glycemic index than fruit juices, sodas, and other sugary drinks, most breads and bread products, white potatoes, white rice, most pastas, fried foods, and refined foods such as potato chips, onion rings, crackers, most granola bars, cookies, cakes, cupcakes (even the designer ones!), and most other sweet treats. Steel cut oatmeal is lower on the glycemic index than rolled oats. Be prepared to wait twenty minutes for it to cook, so plan ahead.

❖ **OLD AND NEW LIST FOR BODYGUARD DAMAGE CONTROL**

If fifty is the new thirty (hallelujah!), and orange is the new black, and if you're bored with those "old/new lists" published on news sites at the end of the year, then check out this actually-relevant-to-your-life-old-new list:

Old	New
Toast/bagels/muffin	A bunch of grapes, half an apple, or one-half cup blueberries, or one slice of high fiber bread
Mashed white potatoes	Mashed cauliflower or sweet potatoes
Cranberry grape juice	Flavored extract water
Cold cereal	Oatmeal or plain yogurt with berries added, along with a handful of nuts (very filling!)

Grits or hash browns	Apple slices or one-half cup guacamole
Mac and cheese or fries	Black beans
Sandwiches	Five-minute nachos (refried beans/guacamole with cilantro/salsa on organic tortilla chips)
Ice cream	Plain (organic) yogurt with one tbsp. honey or organic stevia and lemon extract added
Chocolate cake	Fresh berries with plain yogurt on top (1 tbsp. honey if necessary)
Crackers	Bell pepper strips or carrots
Mayo	Mashed avocado or mustard
Relish	Diced apple and red onions
Salt, MSG seasoned salt	Herbs and spices (rosemary, oregano, basil, dill, parsley, thyme, turmeric). Buy them dried or fresh at the grocery store. You can even grow them…
Store-bought smoothie	Homemade smoothie
Counting calories	Counting carbs and sugars
Counting bad fat	Counting good fat
Ignoring protein	Counting protein
Grocery store	Stopping at the organic market also; ordering non-perishable organic products online
Fiber powder	Fiber-rich foods

❖ AVOIDING SABOTAGE!

In our quest to lose the weight, we often reach for healthy-sounding foods and beverages. They are traps! Don't fall for it. Here are some classic examples:

- **Fruity drinks, store-bought smoothies or restaurant beverages:** Check out the nutritional content of the commercially available smoothie drinks (which shall remain nameless). Likewise, restaurant strawberry lemonades or sweetened teas—the sixteen-ounce glasses with one to two refills? Are you kidding? You'd be better off ordering the apple pie instead.

- **"Healthy" salads:** What's wrong with salad? I can assure you, it's not the lettuce, tomatoes, cucumbers, or onions. The problem is with the dressing, plain and simple. Most dressings are loaded with calories in the form of sugars, unhealthy fats, preservatives, and carbs. An otherwise healthy salad is corrupted when we drown it in a creamy, rich, honey mustard, Vidalia onion, or ranch dressing. For example, most honey mustards have about seven grams of carbs and about seven grams of sugars per serving, which is usually two tablespoons. The problem is that we pour and pour, and if you have ever measured how much you use, it's more like *six to seven tablespoons* of dressing per salad. Now you're looking at twenty-one grams of carbs in the form of sugar just from the dressing. Seriously, when was the last time you used a tablespoon to measure your dressing?

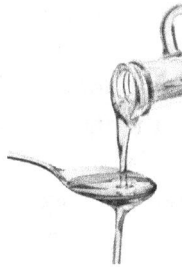

Get the point? Measure your dressing, which should only include vinaigrette or Italian dressing (no exceptions to this rule!). Why vinaigrette? It should be self-evident. It's the "vinaig" part of the word that means it has vinegar in it—one of the best bodyguards going. If you're at home, pull out the tablespoon. If at a restaurant, ask for a tablespoon and ask for the dressing on the side. Do not be embarrassed! Being embarrassed to stand up for ourselves is what landed us in this predicament in the first place.

- **Healthy-sounding snacks:** There is a glut of healthy-sounding protein, breakfast, and granola bars out there. Yet, many are usually high in sugar and loaded with unhealthy preservatives—many of which are endocrine disruptors that hinder your weight-loss efforts. Many of them also contain soybean oil or soy lecithin, which, unless stated otherwise, is likely to be genetically modified.

Healthy-sounding breakfast cereals and other "all natural foods": What does "all natural" mean anyway? Again, judge the product by its nutritional label and ingredient list, and not by its cover—no ifs, ands, or buts about it.

- **Flavored yogurt:** in a word—sugar! Okay, two words: sugar and growth hormones. I only purchase *plain* yogurt and add my own fruit. I take it one step further by buying organic yogurt or at least yogurt from cows that are not given hormones, antibiotics, or steroids.

Swapping soy (non-organic) for meat: Many health advocates believe that cutting red meat out of our diets is the ticket to health and weight loss. While the debate over whether "to be or not to be" a vegetarian rages on, what we choose in the place of meat deserves equal attention. Many of us substitute meat with soy-based, meat-like products. Again, my concerns here are that soy mimics estrogen, and over 90 percent of the soy used in this country is GMO. I highly recommend that you resolve the GMO question for yourself before increasing your consumption of soy, particularly soy that is not organic. Also, make sure you are consuming enough protein, along with your minimum daily iron requirement (I'm talking to the anemics out there . . . you know who you are!). Ultimately, my physician advised that I limit my red meat intake, and I have done so. On those rare occasions when I do eat red meat, I try to avoid meat made from animals that are given antibiotics and artificial growth hormones .

TWO-MINUTE DRILL: STAND UP AND WALK!

CHAPTER 8

Stepping Out

The fruit of the spirit is...self-control...
GALATIANS 5:23

As discussed earlier, I discovered that, on average, I attend nearly thirty cake and ice cream birthday events annually, along with several luncheons, going-away or retirement parties, anniversary parties, brunches, weddings, funerals, church dinners, holiday cookouts, vacation meals, buffets, and the usual let's-just-go-out- meals every year. These food outings add up to around 120–130 out of the 365 days of the year, meaning that well over one-third of my meals involved cake and ice cream, cookies, other rich hors d'oeuvres, appetizers and dishes, lavish meals and/or food prepared by someone else. The point is, our efforts at dropping the weight and regaining our health for the remaining two-thirds of the year are sabotaged by the one-third. So even if you TCB (you know, take care of business) at home, the war on your weight can still be lost the second you step outside your door.

You will discover as I did when attending these events, that when you try to "eat right," the peer pressure to give in and eat the rich, fattening food can be intense. Some people make it their mission to make sure you eat something you don't want, and just saying no doesn't always work. Misery, often unknowingly, really does love company. Accordingly, eating out deserves more than just an honorable mention. It has earned its own chapter.

Now that we are aware of the impact that eating out has on our weight-loss efforts, it's time to learn how to minimize the damage and turn those events to your advantage. Here are seven surefire steps to stop the stepping out slipups.

❖ HOW TO MANAGE EATING OUT

1. **Determine whether you need to attend** all 150–200 events or gatherings in the course of the year. Until you lose the weight, consider setting a personal limit of no more than one "food" outing per week.
2. **Anticipate** the potential damage and prepare in advance.
3. **Fill up with your bodyguards** before you go (fiber, protein snacks, water, raw veggies, and fruit...even oatmeal for goodness' sake! This is war!).
4. **Eat the fibrous, protein, and healthy-fat** items at the event *first*, such as the raw veggies (without the dip), the guacamole, etc.
5. **Sample, don't overdose on the rich carb selections.** If you feel you are falling for the temptation, go ahead and give in *only after* you have filled up with the bodyguards first. Then, take one, no more than two bites. That's it. The idea is that you fill up with the healthy stuff and just *taste* the "tasty" stuff. As a reminder, sugar is addictive. One bite of dessert most certainly will lead to ten more bites.
6. **BYOB.** That's right - bring your own bottle of vinaigrette, vinegar, herbal tea, homemade lemonade, and BPA-free water container. Bring an empty vitamin bottle containing your low-sugar vinaigrette to pour over your veggies if they don't already have it. Have no shame as you BYOB—this is for your health, which should trump the pressure to eat whatever is put before you by someone who does not have to live with your adverse health conditions. There comes a time when you must put *you* first.
7. **Avoid going to a restaurant blind.** Before leaving the office for the going-away luncheon or happy hour, do some recon—access the restaurant's website and preview the nutritional content of its menu items. Compare the nutritional content of the dishes you might want to try, and then decide. Just recently, my family and I went to a popular restaurant for dinner. Before arriving, I researched the nutritional content of the majority of dishes at the restaurant. Are you sitting down? I found a Caesar salad containing over 1200 calories, a chicken dish containing over 1800 calories and 4400 mg of sodium, and a pasta dish containing over 2100 calories, 81 grams of saturated fat, and 144 carbs. As far as possible, don't ever walk into any restaurant "nutritional" sight unseen!

❖ FAB FIVE TIPS FOR TRAVEL AND VACATIONS

For those of you who travel frequently, adding your travel days to the 30–40 percent eating-out equation can push that number closer to 40–50 percent, which makes losing weight even more challenging. Think about it - we rarely factor the total diet damage that job-related and vacation travel bring to the equation.

1. **Plan, plan, plan in advance**: Prior to your scheduled travel, investigate or explore the airport or train station food establishments, along with the nutritional content of the food items on their menus. Also, preview the websites of the restaurants that are in or near your hotel. Select the meals that appear to be the healthiest, and use a search engine to determine what ingredients are used. If you cannot find the information online, call the restaurant. That way, you know in advance where you want to eat. Make a note of what are the least-damaging foods on the menu. If the restaurant selected is outside of your control, don't be afraid to research the nutritional content on your cell phone while ordering. The hindrance is the perception your colleagues have about you. This is a battle you're going to have to win. I Tell them, "I have food allergies" or "I can't eat soy." Visiting relatives? If you know that cousin Bubba's wife, Betty, fries everything in sight and wouldn't know a fresh vegetable if it hit her on the head, be prepared to fill up with your bodyguards. Insist on going to the grocery store on the way from the airport. Tell them you need some nasal spray (hey, it's all I could think of!). Buy your organic veggies, soy-free salad dressing (better yet, make your own!), fruit, and snacks to keep with you at the house.

2. **Aim to maintain while on vacation.** You may have found a way to lose weight on vacation (because you drank the water!), but usually I am not that fortunate. The end game for me while on vacation is simply not to gain. Again, it's about damage control. Deploy your bodyguards every day, and make sure you walk your ten thousand steps—that's right, the pedometer does *not* vacay when you're on vacay, not when you have to lose fifty pounds, sorry. By the way, don't forget to take the pedometer off before stepping into the hot tub (not saying I forgot...).

   Also, forget about the liquid lunches—you know, two piña coladas to chase the five-thousand-calorie breakfast buffet meal. Bring this book with you and read it on the plane. If you must indulge, do NOT drink or eat any uber-sugary or mega-carb ANYTHING on an empty stomach! Hip-hop moguls do not leave their bodyguards at home while they vacation and neither should you.

3. **Bring your own food.** What? Isn't that going too far? It depends. If you are serious about controlling what you eat and do not want to be at the mercy of food establishments, you should bring nonperishables or perishables packed in cooler packs. Items such as oatmeal packets, nuts, stevia packets, fruit, salads, and guacamole can travel right along with you. I even bring my frozen organic burritos and cook them in my hotel room's kitchen.

4. **Consider staying at hotels with kitchens.** Doing so allows you to prepare your own meals. Bring food to heat up in your room, and keep your perishables in the refrigerator. *Warning*: some hotels send minibar commandos to storm your room the second you open the touch-sensor minibar door. So you might want to inquire in advance about using the minibar. Seriously, they will bill you for uneaten snacks!

5. **Have the hotel stock your refrigerator.** These days, several hotels are willing to stock your hotel refrigerator in advance for you. Or, find out what nearby grocery or specialty stores will deliver healthy food products to your hotel for a small fee. It may be worth it if your travel is extended. You can always research organic personal chefs who also will deliver dinner to your hotel for a small fee. The world as we know it has changed.

❖ HOLIDAYS, FEASTS, BIRTHDAYS, AND OTHER BIG GATHERINGS

Is she about to talk about...SOUL FOOD?
Excuse me? Do we have a problem? It depends. When we gather for potluck church dinners, family barbecues and dinners, even Thanksgiving or Christmas, we make sure that all the possible meats are covered—pork ribs, burgers, hamburgers, pork chops, hot dogs with bleached white bread buns, *fried* fish, chitterlings or pig's feet, fried chicken, and more fried chicken, ham, etc. Then, we cover the carbs—the cornbread, rolls, candied yams, rice, corn on the cob, corn pudding, potato salad, mashed potatoes, mac and cheese, and pasta salad. Did I miss anything? Usually, the token veggies are overcooked green beans or collards. Rarely is there a salad or other fresh veggie or fruit at the table.

Healthy or unhealthy?

Soul food, down-home cooking or southern cuisine, like any other cuisine, is not good or bad in and of itself. Instead, we make it unhealthy by how we prepare it, how much of it we eat, and which foods we choose to eat. For example, kidney, navy, lima and black beans, and of course, black-eyed peas used to be staples in the soul-food repertoire. Collard and mustard greens, kale, Brussels sprouts, cauliflower, cabbage, and broccoli also are part of the soul food/southern cuisine experience, but we rarely cook five or six of these savory dishes as part of our feasts. No, we throw in one of these dishes for good measure—usually green beans from a can (you know it's true!), and we stock up on the heavy carbohydrates, meats, sweets and sweet drinks. It is time to readjust the family feast food pyramid to elevate the greens and other vegetables, along with the fish dishes described below, to the top.

Fish: not just for the fish fry

Fish is another category of "meat" that is considered down home or soul food, and there are all sorts—salmon, trout, whiting, red snapper, porgies, perch, cod, and bass. In fact, our grandparents caught and cooked many of these fishes. These days, we overload on the red meats, many of which are filled with hormones and antibiotics, unlike in days gone by. Also, many are derived from animals that are fed food that is genetically modified or overly *pesticized*. (Did I just create a word? Please contact *Webster's* to add it to the dictionary next year.) Ultimately, I learned to reduce my consumption of red meat because I don't want antibiotics for dinner, and because I no longer work off the fat the way my grandparents did. The red meat has been replaced with many of the fishes mentioned above.

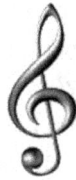

On the fifth day of Christmas, my true love gave to me:
FIVE...PORK...RIBS!
Four buttered rolls
Three cured hams
Two turkey wings
And a slice of seven-layer cake!

Sorry to bust anyone's bubble, but gone are the days when we can eat three to four pieces of red meat of any kind, five to six servings of carbohydrates, two rolls or slices of cornbread, two to three desserts, along with sixteen ounces of punch, lemonade, soda, or worse—egg nog—all in one sitting and think there will be no health consequences. This is where self-control must take the reins. The idea is not to have one of each of everything but to have a variety from which to choose. Our advancing age, slowing metabolisms, health conditions, and sedentary lifestyles simply do not allow for the usual smorgasbords anymore.

Somewhere, someone said, "Well, we're going to die of something so we might as well eat all we want." That misplaced mantra became a license for eating anything and everything our bellies could hold. What they forgot to tell us is that the ensuing years will be filled with knee pain, back pain, arthritis, indigestion, acid reflux, diabetes, amputations, strokes, cardiovascular disease, prescription drugs for high blood pressure, high sugar, high cholesterol, migraines, and so on and so on. Yes, we are all going to die of something, but there's no need to speed up the process; and there's no need to be miserable in the meantime.

A new approach...

These days, when cooking the feast, my husband and I take the opportunity to lower the glycemic load of nearly every dish we prepare. First, we make sure that the beverages contain little to no sugar. That's right, it is lazy-girl lemonade, limeade, or flavored tea with a tad bit of coconut sugar, honey, or organic stevia. Mashed potatoes? I usually swap cauliflower for around half of the potatoes. Yams are always on the menu, but instead of sugar, again, we use organic stevia and vanilla flavoring, with lots of cinnamon and nutmeg. We always serve salad and offer soy-free vinaigrettes only. Finally, we usually prepare at least two to three other green vegetables such as Brussels sprouts, broccoli, collard greens, or kale. Stuffing? Yes, but homemade from slices of organic high-protein/high-fiber bread. You get the point. It is all about preserving taste while cutting sugar and bad fat, and lowering the glycemic load...It is about damage control!

Last, and by no means least, are...

❖ DESSERTS!

Desserts are so highly prized that they get their own table! Need I say more? Red velvet cake, banana pudding, bread pudding, rice pudding, double chocolate cake, sundaes, brownies, chocolate chip cookies, strawberry short-cake, cheesecake, upscale and designer (though still sugary) cupcakes, apple pie, peach cobbler, and blueberry pie. And each of us gets a slice of EACH! Did I miss anything? Oh, how can I forget...ice cream. The sugar content can range from 72 grams for a slice of chocolate cake with one-half cup of ice cream to over 100 grams for a Sundae. Then something called "itis" sets in. I prefer to call it insulin resistance. To make matters worse, instead of walking for thirty minutes after that carbohydrate-and-sugar-feeding frenzy, we sit and sit for hours. That's all I'm going to say on that subject.

Dessert Alternatives

First, let me confess that I had a sliver (or two) of my cousin's chocolate raspberry cheesecake at Thanksgiving this year. At least I drank an ounce of apple- cider vinegar in a glass of water (my bodyguard) *before* eating the cheesecake! Thanksgiving is tough, I admit. That said, feel free to eat low-sugar, higher-protein/fiber dessert alternatives for the rest of the year. Here are my favorites:

1. Enjoy Life Mixed Berry or Chocolate Bars
2. Cascadian Farms Organic Protein Bars
3. Homemade granola with organic coconut ice cream
4. Berry parfait (layer fresh berries, plain Greek yogurt mixed with stevia and one-half teaspoon lemon extract, and organic chocolate or granola bar crumble)
5. Ambrosia with fruit and coconut
6. One-half cup organic coconut ice cream with berries
7. Fresh fruit
8. **No dessert** (what a thought!)

❖ **REMEMBER, IT'S ABOUT DAMAGE CONTROL!**

As a recap, here are some things to do before you leave home for the feast or party:

- Drink two to three glasses of water, with the juice of a half of lemon or lime.
- Eat a handful of nuts twenty minutes before eating anything else.
- Eat a large salad, with vinaigrette dressing.

- Have a big bowl of oatmeal.
- Drink a plain yogurt smoothie (one cup yogurt, berries) in the car.
- Avoid "carb bigamy." Instead of choosing *all* the carbs at a meal, choose *between* carbs. If you decide to have the punch, then resist the chips and cake; if you decide on the mac and cheese, then resist the rolls; if you decide to have cake, make it a sliver that *you* slice. I promise you, others will cut it large and you will eat all of it, so cut it yourself. Then, toss the frosting from your sliver and drink water.
- MOVE! MOVE! MOVE! Stand up and start moving; take a walk outside or sneak in a few side leg kicks. The last thing I want to do is to eat way too much and then sit for hours. Do whatever it takes to move. After thirty minutes, stand and move about again. Note: the more family and friends who partner with you in your *JustForMeDiet* journey, the more people who'll walk with you after the meal, bring healthier dishes to the gathering, and encourage you to eat more healthy food.

CHAPTER 9

Lose The Liquid Pounds!

I discipline my body and keep it under control.
I CORINTHIANS 9:27

M any individuals who need to lose weight do not realize that they are *drinking* a hefty portion of their daily calories, sugars, and carbs. We drink hundreds of calories and dozens of sugar and carb grams on a daily basis just from our sodas, juices, "healthy" smoothies, the sugar and creamer in our coffees, lattes, frappuccinos, sugared teas, specialty waters, and of course, fruity cocktails, wine, and beer. We are drinking liquid pounds.

Those carbs and sugar grams can add up to twenty to thirty pounds gained...or lost (that's up to *you*) over the course of a year. Our intake of liquid pounds is a secret saboteur, but as discussed below, this is one of the easiest adjustments to make. A note of caution: if you think diet sodas are the answer to your weight-loss dilemma, think again. A recent study found that people who drink diet sodas actually consume more calories than those who do not drink diet sodas. Not only that, but another recent study suggested that the artificial sweeteners in these beverages are now linked to diabetes and belly fat. So, let's take a minute to look at what we've been drinking that has packed on our pounds—and find delicious and healthy alternatives.

❖ SUGARY-SWEET STUMBLING BLOCKS

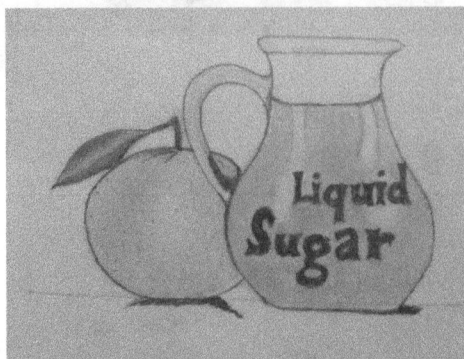

Fruit juices, including orange juice

Yes, I know, orange juice is the morning's sacred cow. As we learned earlier, a twelve-ounce glass of OJ has *thirty-three grams of sugar*. Does that sentence need repeating...again? Thirty-three grams of sugar. In Spanish, that's *thirty-three gramos de azucar*! If you eliminate that morning drink, you just might drop another eight to ten pounds during the year.

Cranberry juice has about thirty-two grams of sugar per eight-ounce glass. Again, with that amount of sugar, you've exceeded your sugar intake for the day, before you've taken your first bite of food. If you're diabetic, you have exceeded your sugar intake for the day. Moreover, most drinking glasses or tumblers in our kitchen cabinets are twelve-ounce glasses, so if you fill the glass up, you really are drinking forty grams of sugar. And if you refill that glass, well...you do the math!

Coffee

First and foremost, *frappés*, *mochas*, "*machis*" (my nickname for macchiatos), and all hard-to-spell coffee drinks have to go. Period. When you see the sugar content chart, you'll understand why. There is no room on the *JustForMeDiet* for any member of that extended family.

Your eyes see mochaccino...but your fat cells
see sugar cubes in a fancy glass!

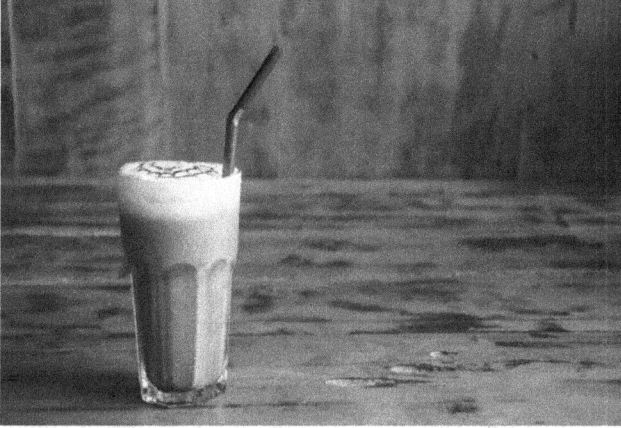

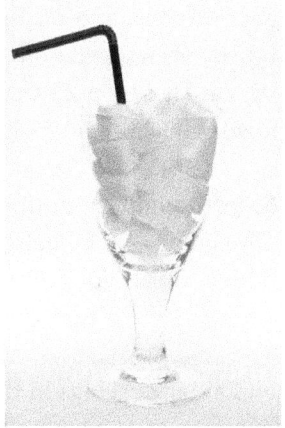

Even if you just drink plain 'ole coffee, you probably maintain an extra five to ten pounds per year just from the sugar and heavy creamers, whether in powder or in liquid form. As I'm sure you have discovered by now in this guide, the road to health and to becoming svelte is through substitutions. For example, a cup of coffee with three packets of sugar (or so) adds up to forty-five calories and fifteen sugar grams...Ugh! The creamer is thirty-five calories per tablespoon. But, really now, have you ever actually measured a tablespoon of creamer? Do you realize how little that is? The point is, whether at the coffee house or in my own kitchen, I had NEVER pulled out the measuring spoon to measure my creamer. Hmm, where did I put my measuring spoon? Really? I just POUR!

"Ma'am, would you like some coffee with your sugar and cream?"

I finally measured how much cream and sugar I had been scooping and pouring and realized it was around five tablespoons! That's over two hundred calories for the creamer and sugar, which for one year is around 73,000 calories. Divide that by thirty-five hundred calories (3500 calories = one pound) and you get over *twenty pounds*! I also realized that the liquid creamer contained six grams of sugar per tablespoon, which totaled thirty grams of sugar from the creamer and another fifteen from the sugar, or about forty-five grams of sugar before I even started the day. Moment of silence...

Again, although counting calories was not part of my weight-loss journey, eliminating the obvious high-sugar/high-calorie foods and beverages were part of the weight-loss strategy. It's that easy. By eliminating all creamers, switching to almond milk, and nixing the sugar, I dropped forty-five grams of sugar per day. I probably knocked off at least fifteen pounds just by changing how I drank my coffee! These days, I alternate between almond milk and two ounces of organic low-fat milk.

Store-bought smoothie drinks
OMG! They look healthy enough. The products' labels claim there is no sugar added, but if you look at the nutrition label you will see these store-bought smoothies contain upward of twenty-seven grams of sugar PER SERVING! The sugar is natural, but it is still sugar. Moreover, there just might be three and a half servings in the container. That's three and a half times the amount of sugar you need for the day. If one serving contains thirty grams of sugar, at three and a half servings per container, you will drink 105 grams of sugar before you finish. Therefore, I never, ever buy these beverages.

Lemonades and flavored teas
How many of us have gone out to a restaurant for lunch or dinner and ordered the strawberry lemonade or the golfer's lemonade/tea drink? Think about it: the glass is huge, around twenty ounces, and refills are free. The twenty ounces of strawberry lemonade just cost you seventy-four grams of sugar, and that's before the first refill. Just say no and drink water with lemon instead.

Cocktails
I was almost kicked out of a lazy river in Aruba when I mentioned that piña coladas have as many calories as a double cheeseburger. The other lazy-river queens did not want to be reminded of that. But we need to be reminded. Consider that the average calorie content of a twelve-ounce glass of piña colada is 655, around eighty-five carbs and eighty-four sugars. By the way, most hurricane glasses are twenty ounces. Add just one more piña colada and you have 168 grams of sugar. Going to the resort's fitness center for a thirty-minute run later on in the day will not undo the sugar spike and fat storage you just triggered with those cocktails. Guess what? That's not the

worst part. As if the sugar itself wasn't bad enough, when mixed with alcohol, it spells double trouble for your diet. I recently read that alcohol slows our metabolism by around seventy percent. The alcohol slows fat burning at a time when you need fat to be burned, given all the sugar you are drinking! The chart below identifies the sugar content of many beverages we drink day and night. It is a short list of some shockers:

BEVERAGE	SUGARS
1. McDonald's McCafe Chocolate Shake (22 oz.)	120 g (and 850 cal.!)
2. Orange Julius Triple Berry Smoothie (large)	105 g
3. Wendy's Strawberry Lemonade (large)	84 g
4. Minute Maid Lemonade (20 oz.)	67 g
5. Coke (20 oz.)	65 g
6. McDonalds Oreo McFlurry (12 oz.)	64 g
7. Starbucks Caramel Frappuccino Blended Coffee (16 oz.)	64 g
8. StarbucksWhite Hot Chocolate (grande)	62 g
9. Jamba Juice Sunrise Banana Berry (16 oz.)	59 g
10. Starbucks Iced White Chocolate Mocha (grande)	55 g
11. Naked Berry Blast (15.2 oz.)	54 g
12. Apple juice (12 oz.)	42 g
13. Snapple Peach Tea (16 oz.)	39 g
14. Orange juice (12 oz.)	33 g
15. Vitamin Water Energy Drink (20 oz.)	32 g

LEST WE FORGET...COCKTAILS

16. Piña Colada (12 oz.)	84 g
17. Margarita (6 oz.)	24 g
18. Mojito (6 oz.)	18 g

Moment of silence...

Now that we have dismissed all of the *JustForMeDiet* saboteurs from the table, let's look at low- or no-sugar alternatives...

❖ **SIPS FROM SEVEN SEAS!**

1. **Water:** I know it doesn't taste like much (hmmm...that's because it's tasteless), but it can't be beat. We've heard that we're supposed to have eight eight-ounce glasses of water per day. Herbal tea can count toward that magic number. I also have heard that your water intake in ounces should be half of your body weight. Some people swear by a gallon of water per day. My experience is that there are general guidelines that need to be adjusted to match your environment and/or health condition. If your water intake has been restricted for medical reasons, please adhere to those restrictions. If you are working outside in the sweltering heat all day long, or if you have a fever, you probably need more than eight glasses. If you drink three to four mugs of decaffeinated herbal tea per day, you probably do not need an additional eight glasses of water. Generally, eight or so glasses per day (water and unsweetened herbal tea) is sufficient for me. You might only need six glasses. Your body has a way of telling you when you're not getting enough water. Clues are dizziness, excessive hunger, thirst, constipation, swollen feet, headaches, faintness, etc.

Many people tell me they just don't like the taste of water, or they hate having to get up from their desks to go to the bathroom all day. Some people "forget" to drink water. But consider this: According to the CDC[xxix], drinking water will:

1. Keep your temperature normal
2. Lubricate and cushion joints
3. Protect your spinal cord and other sensitive tissues
4. Rid your body of waste through urination, perspiration, and bowel movements

According to Authority Nutrition[xxx], drinking water will:

5. Increase the number of calories you burn for up to ninety minutes
6. Make you burn about ninety-six more calories per day if you drink at least sixty-eight ounces
7. Help reduce hunger, and according to one study, drop up to forty-four percent more weight over twelve weeks if at least seventeen ounces are consumed thirty minutes before meals

Also, keep in mind that we often reach for food when in fact we're just thirsty. I found that drinking water satisfied my thirst and my hunger. Water also gives me more energy, and it also helps me to think more clearly.

****

JustForMeDiet Tip: I hate water, so how do I drink more?

- *Place a full glass by your bed at night; cover with a napkin; drink immediately after your early morning weigh-in.*
- *Drink a glass when you get to work.*
- *Drink one glass every two hours while at work and one before leaving for home.*
- *Drink one to two glasses, thirty minutes before dinner.*
- *Fill your forty-ounce stainless-steel water bottle with purified water at home before leaving for work in the morning, and do not leave work until you have finished drinking all of it.*

****

2. **Water with lemon or lime:** Yes, that's more like it. This beverage deserves its own paragraph, distinct from water alone. In fact, there are so many natural flavorings you can add to water to transform that tasteless, odorless liquid into a tasty beverage. This is where the cute juice extractor comes in. You just grab the lemon or lime, cut it in half, put one-half in the squeezer, squeeze into the water, and put the other half in the fridge. It's that simple. If you really want to spice things up, put a couple of mint leaves in the glass. You can even add a packet of stevia to create what I call...

3. **Lazy-girl lemonade or limeade:** I also call this beverage the "el-emonator." The lazy-girl lemonade eliminates sugar and calories. Just use your lemon/lime juice squeezer to squeeze the juice of half a lemon or lime into a glass, add one to two teaspoons of organic stevia, and then fill with water. Stir and you're done. Fresh squeezed lemonade or limeade by the glass. It's that simple—it's tasty, healthy, sugar free, carb free, fat free, and guilt free! You will never grow tired of this beverage. If you prefer not to use the stevia, for just a few sugar grams, you can add a tbsp. of coconut sugar or organic raw sugar.

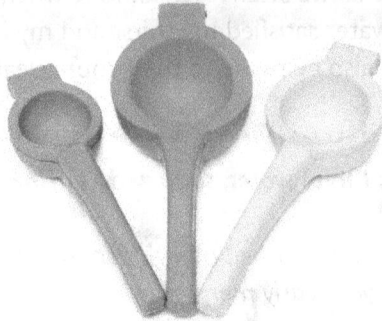

4. **Strawberry basil or tart cherry basil lemonade:** This is my all-time favorite. Just toss some strawberries (or one ounce of tart cherry juice), a few basil leaves, the juice of half a lemon, either one or two packets of organic stevia, or one tablespoon of honey and ice into your blender and blend away. This beverage is a game changer!

5. **Juice and spice extracts**: Just squeeze a few drops of these extracts into your water and voila—you have a great-tasting beverage containing no sugar or sugar substitute. Try lemon and lime, ginger, and pomegranate. Many of these tasty extracts contain no sugar, calories, fat, carbs or artificial ingredients, and they are high in antioxidants. Moreover, many brands need no refrigeration, so you can carry them in your purse or backpack. You can keep one at work and take one with you when you go out to eat. Yes, add it to your restaurant water. Do *not* feel guilty about *not* paying money for a soda or a strawberry lemonade (dozens of sugar grams) at a restaurant. Check out this website to see one of the brands I like best: (**www.Pureinventions.com**).

6. **Iced herbal tea:** Purchase your favorite box of herbal tea from an array of herbal tea brands and flavors. Some flavors—cinnamon, mints, berries, orange spice, and chai - are so tasty that adding a sweetener will ruin the good flavor. Brew the tea, add the ice and a mint leaf.

7. **Veggie juice:** Juice your favorite veggies, whether kale, broccoli, cabbage, parsley, carrots, cucumbers, with an apple to cut the bitter flavor. When juicing apples, berries, and other highly-sugared fruits together, keep in mind that you might be making homemade liquid sugar. I advise that you juice the veggies and add no more than one sugary fruit.

❖ SIPS WHEN STEPPING OUT

Most of us spend the majority of our time outside of our homes. This is where we eat most of our food, and it's where we drink—or don't drink—most of our water. Like meal planning, I plan for beverages. Not only must we control and eliminate the high-sugar and high-carbohydrate beverages while we're away from home, but we must also find ways to replace them with healthy beverages, including water, the "elemonator," and other beverages. How do we accomplish this when outside the home? Here are some ideas:

- I carry a forty-ounce stainless-steel water bottle with me. I fill it up in the morning from my refrigerator's filtered water. As long as I drink all of the water before I return home, I know I've consumed at least forty of the sixty-four ounces of water I need for the day.
- When eating at restaurants, I ask for water with lemon or lime. I might even add a packet of organic stevia from the stash I keep in my purse. Again, feel free to add a few flavored extract drops to the water to create a beverage.
- Consider buying a filter to install on the sink in your kitchen. I know what you're thinking—pricey, right? I have an idea: instead of buying individual gifts for Christmas, buy one gift for the whole family—the water filter. Granted, your family probably won't speak to you for a while, but they'll forget all about it by spring.

TWO MINUTE DRILL!

CHAPTER 10

Move It!

But they that wait on the Lord shall renew their strength...they shall run and not be weary, and they shall walk and not faint.
ISAIAH 40:31

Let me get right to the point. Sitting all day and all evening is probably one of the top-three greatest threats to our health, afflicting both young and old. Everyone knows that smoking is deadly. Everyone knows to just say no to drugs. Yet, we all have underestimated the danger presented by sitting all day, and the correlation between sitting all day and diabetes, obesity, even cancer - hence, the term "sitting disease." Recently, health authorities have been sounding that alarm. The alarming fact is that most Americans sit all day at work, only to come home and sit all evening in front of the television.

X-ray of the Sitting Disease!

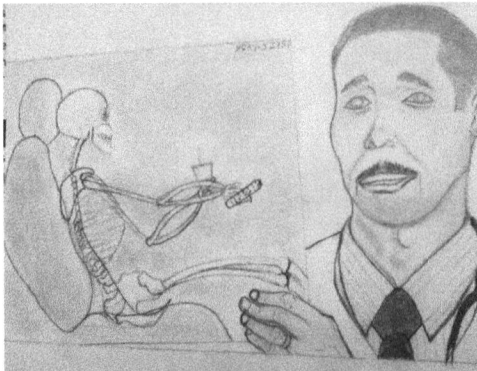

❖ HOW DID WE GET HERE?

Decades ago, before the office high-rise and computer workstation became the altars where Americans worshipped all day, our grandparents were not sitting in front of computers and televisions all day. Grandpa and grandma never saw the inside of a fitness center yet they were slimmer and trimmer than today's middle-aged Americans. They also didn't suffer from diabetes and obesity as does this current generation. Instead, they worked in fields, farms, and factories (blasphemy, right?). They came home and cleaned the house, repaired furniture, and even made furniture. They cut their own lawns, raked their own leaves, and shoveled their own snow. They even trimmed the hedges manually (scary, I know!) They didn't need the gym and they didn't pay personal trainers. No Zumba, spin classes, or Pilates for Nana. Instead, Nana actually stood up and walked to the TV to turn the channel, hand washed clothes, hung them to dry, hand washed and dried dishes, walked to the post office, washed windows and walls…Are you getting the point?

Our activity levels moved from sixty to zero in two decades.

Now we have motorized mowers, electric hedge trimmers, leaf blowers, and snow blowers. Or we contract for lawn service and hire landscapers. The laundry room is now on the bedroom level, so we do not have to trek up and down the stairs with heavy laundry baskets. Who needs the gym when you can do laundry for two to three hours? When was the last time you raked leaves with a rake? Talk about getting your heart rate up! We sit all day at the computer, and then we go home to sit all evening in front of the television. Those sitting hours add up to around ten to twelve hours per day.

Right about now you're thinking: *Is this woman suggesting that we ditch the office job and head for green acres (wasn't that a TV show?)* Calm down. Let's not get carried away. Nor am I suggesting that you throw away your washing machine because I most certainly still have mine. I'm simply saying we must learn to reincorporate unstructured physical activity and movement, even house and yard work, into our lives every day. Making that adjustment just might extend your life.

❖ WHY WE MUST STAND UP and MOVE!

According to the CDC,

"Prolonged sitting time (as a specific instance of sedentary behavior), independent of physical activity, has emerged as a risk factor for various negative

health outcomes. Study results have demonstrated associations of prolonged sitting time with premature mortality; chronic diseases such as cardiovascular disease, diabetes, and cancer; metabolic syndrome; and obesity. In contrast, breaks in prolonged sitting time have been correlated with beneficial metabolic profiles among adults, suggesting that frequent breaks in sedentary activity may explain lower health risk related to waist circumference, Body Mass Index (BMI), triglyceride levels, and two-hour plasma glucose levels." [xxxi]

Translation: by sitting all day, we stay fat and sick, and we shorten our lifespan. By breaking up the long-seated stretches, we can turn things around.

The CDC is not the only organization sounding the alarm on the deadly effects of sitting all day long. Just go to your favorite search engine and research "sitting and mortality," "sitting and cancer" or "sitting and diabetes." Articles from the CDC, journals published by the National Institutes for Health (NIH) and other health organizations will surface—read them all! The results will shock you. You will discover that sitting all day will *significantly* raise your risk of those deadly diseases identified by the CDC. The worst part is that everyone believes that going to the gym or exercise class for an hour three days per week will offset the effects of sitting all day. Those same studies will prove that myth to be wrong! One hour of working out per day will <u>not</u> offset the adverse impact to our health caused by sitting for the rest of the day. You need to see this for yourself. Return to your favorite search engine and search "sitting all day" and "exercise" and "offset" to find the eye-opening truth that de-bunks the myth that my spin class will undo the damage done by sitting the rest of the day.

Please share this information with everyone you know who regularly sits all day long. In fact, even while writing this book, I was conscious of sitting too long and stood up at least every thirty minutes to walk or bounce on my mini-trampoline for a couple of minutes.

What a difference two minutes make!

When people ask me to tell them what I did to lose the weight, I tell them, "I clipped a pedometer to my skirt or slacks and moved all day long." Here's why: A study measured the blood sugar spikes and insulin resistance of individuals who were sedentary for seven hours against those who stood every twenty minutes to walk on a treadmill for just two minutes during the last five hours of the seven-hour period. The individuals who never rose from their desks experienced sugar spikes and an increase in insulin all day, *while the group that rose every twenty minutes for just two minutes experienced no sugar spikes or insulin resistance.* A third group stood every twenty minutes to jog on the treadmill for two minutes, yet there was no statistically significant difference between their blood sugar and insulin levels and the levels of the group that walked. *See* "Too Much Sitting: Health Risks of Sedentary Behavior and Opportunities for Change," President's Council on Fitness, Sports and Nutrition, Series 13, Number 3, December 2012.

Now you know the origin of the "two-minute drill!"

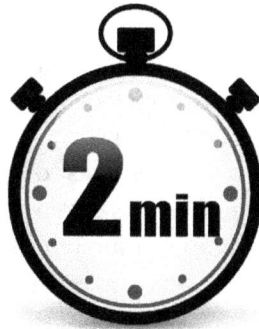

Implement the "two-minute drill."
Since the study shows that standing and walking for two minutes every twenty minutes will reduce blood sugar spikes and insulin resistance, we must plan to stand up every twenty to thirty minutes during the day and in the evening when we get home. For those of you who are glued to the computer for hours at a time, set an alarm to remind yourself to stand up and perform two minutes of leg kicks or to walk around your building with something to read. This is legitimate work time as long as you are reading work materials. If you must, talk to your supervisor about the need to stand and move more often.

LET'S GET BUSY MOVING!
Health experts recommend that we engage in at least thirty minutes of physical activity per day to reduce our risk of cancer, cardiovascular diseases, diabetes, and obesity, among other conditions. To give yourself a fighting chance in this weight-loss journey, you must rise from that chair, that sofa, that bed, or move away from that television and computer every twenty to thirty minutes and move—*for just two minutes*. The good news is that you don't have to run around your building for

those two minutes. You don't have to join the gym, you don't have to run a marathon, and you don't even need to pay a personal trainer. You do need to move more—a lot more. Below are some suggestions for moving more.

Have some fun bouncing on a mini trampoline
Bouncing on a mini trampoline or rebounder is a very low-impact way to move; it elevates the heart rate, burns calories, and stimulates the lymphatic system all at the same time. Bouncing is fun, helps tone muscles throughout the body, boosts your immune system, stimulates the lymphatic system, and lets you get your inner child on. This easy to use device is portable, and you can even remove the legs and load it into the backseat or trunk of your car for road trips. The price ranges from forty dollars and up, and you can find them at sporting goods stores. I spent sixty-nine dollars on the one I currently own. Believe me when I say this is the easiest way to watch TV while working out, particularly during the winter when it is dark and cold outside. You can even pick up a couple of hand weights to hold while you bounce to burn even more calories. Sisters, for some serious cardio and arm work, you can pretend you are turning a double-dutch rope while jumping double-dutch style on the mini-trampoline. Just a few minutes every thirty minutes will make a huge difference.

Keep in mind, this device requires balance, and if you are balance challenged, many mini-trampolines are sold with a stability bar to hold on to. Bounce while watching your favorite show or put on some music and jump away!

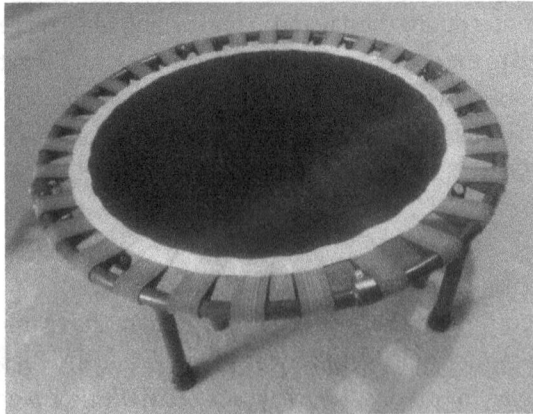

NOTE: Consult your physician before starting any new form of physical activity, particularly if you are balance-challenged.

Do "deskercises"

Deskercises will help you tone and even build muscle without having to go to the gym. I suggest you start slowly and build up to three sets of fifteen to twenty reps of each exercise. I break them up and mix them up. I might stand up to do the three sets of arm rotations and get back to work. Mid-afternoon, I will do the leg kicks while on a telecom, and later in the afternoon, I might do two sets of wall pushups. Each set took two or three minutes. You can find ideas online for exercises you can do while sitting or standing at your desk or workstation, and YouTube videos demonstrate how to do those exercises. Feel free to create a routine with the exercises below or create your own list...

Arms

- Arm rotations
- Arm curls with hand weight
- Wall and desk pushups
- Tricep desk dips
- Overhead arm scissors
- Working with resistance bands

Legs

- Side leg kicks
- Front to back leg kicks
- Squats
- Seated leg raises
- Seated leg scissors
- Walking or jogging in place for 2-3 minutes (feel free to lift those hand weights)

Whole body/waist

- Torso twists
- Side bends
- Jumping jacks
- Dancing!
- Squat jumps

Burn some calories on a mini-exercise peddler

I used one of these devices to help rehabilitate my shoulder following rotator cuff surgery. They are useful for arm exercises and you can slip this device under your desk at work and peddle away calories while you work. In fact, a 200-pound person can burn over 350 calories per hour with this hideaway device. Not bad, huh? Can't you see yourself typing away at the computer while revving your metabolism and burning calories at the same time? It simply can't be beat!

Get stepping on a mini stair-stepper

Yes, another *mini*, but fear not! This device does not cost that much (fifty dollars and up) and some come with resistance bands. You can store your mini stepper in your office and burn real calories with it. A 200-pound person can burn over 500 calories per hour on this mini-device. Should you stair-step for one full hour in your office? Probably not, unless there's a shower stall down the hall; however, just a two or three minute stair-step break can stimulate fat burning and stabilize blood sugar.

Create an oldies playlist and dance!

Create a playlist of your favorite songs. At least once or twice a week, get busy dancing! Dance while you clean, dance while you cook, and dance during commercials. Thirty minutes of singing and dancing your favorite songs will burn fat, and boost your metabolism, mood and immunity. So, get busy dancing!

****

JUSTFORME TIP: I Am a Receptionist or
Therapist and Must Sit All Day.

> *If sitting all day is an absolute must, make the best of the personal time you do have. Walk around your house or apartment for five to ten minutes in the morning before you leave; use your two fifteen-minute breaks to stand up and walk around the building, weather permitting. Stand up and do a few leg kicks, even if you are chained to that workspace. Create your "deskercise" routine and do a few of them every hour—two minutes worth. Take the scenic route to the bathroom, and be sure to walk during your thirty-minute lunch break. If you must eat during those thirty minutes, walk for twenty and eat for ten. If you're a therapist, the sessions usually last fifty minutes or so. Squeeze in your two-minute drill between clients. Use the mini-peddler while sitting or the mini-stair stepper during your breaks. When you get home, make sure you are moving throughout the evening.*

****

Adopt often overlooked ways to move

Put on your pedometer, the electronic step counter, or your cell phone pedometer (there's something for techies and non-techies), and start stepping.
Aim for taking *at least* ten thousand steps staggered throughout the day—
that's about five miles. Feel free to take more than ten thousand steps. *Move
all day long.* I aim to reach the first one thousand steps before leaving home,
and the pedometer measures my progress as the day wears on. Remember
lose the lunch crowd? The idea is to use that time to walk—walk around your
building; walk to the mall, and bring the lunch crowd with you; walk inside of
an empty conference room while reading work documents; and walk up and
down the stairs at work. You also can walk on the treadmill or around your
house.

The outcome you want will not happen without declaring *war* on your sedentary life. We *must* move on a regular basis—preferably, aim to take four or five
activity breaks in your day. Below are dozens of ideas for how to walk and move
more often:

➤ *Morning*

- Upon rising, stretch for one to two minutes, and then walk around
  for three to five minutes.
- If you drive to work, park as far from your office as possible to add a
  few extra steps per day. They add up.
- If you are on the train, stand while waiting for the train and, if not
  weighted down with stuff, try to stand during most if not all of the
  ride. If possible, walk while on the escalator. Better yet, take the stairs
  from time to time.
- Walk one flight of stairs before getting on the elevator at work, or get
  off one floor early and walk the last flight of stairs.

➤ *Workplace*

- At lunchtime, walk *instead of* eating out. At midday, walk to a café
  to buy a cup of herbal tea with lemon. During the winter, locate the
  closest mall to walk indoors during your lunch break.
- Once or twice per day, walk to another floor to use the restroom.

- Stand up and talk during conference calls.
- Schedule your teleconferences throughout the day so that you have opportunities in both the morning and the afternoon to stand up while talking.
- Stand up and walk around the office while you read work materials.
- Go to an empty conference room to accomplish this "reading while walking" movement.
- Ask your human resource professional for a standing computer work station for alternating between sitting and standing.
- Stand up and march in place for two minutes. Do twenty leg kicks per leg while standing.
- Set your phone alarm or your computer to remind you to stand, stretch, and walk every thirty minutes.
- Drink more water. Doing so will send you to the bathroom more often. Granted, many people complain about having to get up to go to the bathroom, but now we know we actually need to stand up and walk more often.
- Instead of emailing your colleagues, get up and walk to them.

➤ *Evening*

- Stand and walk while talking on the phone. Loop the dining room, kitchen, living room, or den. You can walk inside your apartment or house with the same success. Just keep walking.
- If you work on the computer at home, again, take a break every thirty minutes. Consider placing your laptop on an elevated surface to work while standing.
- Check your pedometer when you get home. If you are under seven thousand steps, begin to walk about, even while you cook. I'll put a pot on the stove and then walk around while waiting for the water to boil. The idea is to keep moving!
- Fire your housekeeper and clean your own house.
- March in place and do standing crunches while brushing your teeth.
- Do one or two strenuous chores two nights per week. Make sure the job takes at least thirty minutes. Your house will thank you.

➢ *Television time*

  ○ Stand up during commercials and telephone calls and walk your floors. I probably should include the stairs more than I do. Oh, well. You set the example for me!
  ○ Hop onto the mini trampoline and get busy jumping! Don't wait to change clothes—get some steps or jumps in the minute you walk in the door. Don't forget to grab your one or two pound hand weights.
  ○ Get peddling with your mini exercise peddler while watching your favorite show.
  ○ Turn the channel to the music station during commercials and dance to whatever song is playing.

➢ *Grocery store*

  ○ Park far away from the store (feel free to ignore this tip if it happens to be dark, raining, icing, snowing, or sleeting, if you happen to be in the middle of a hurricane or a tornado, or if you are pregnant).
  ○ Walk the cart to your car and return it all the way to the store (not to the cart corral). Cha-ching goes the pedometer.
  ○ Walk all the aisles at least once to increase your steps, and then begin shopping. Big discount stores are great for walking. Make sure you have on your walking shoes.
  ○ Use the smaller cart if possible. The grocery stores actually increased the size of their carts to get us to buy more food—and it worked!

➢ *During kid chauffeur time*

There is a common condition suffered by hundreds of thousands of mothers and fathers across this great land called "chauffeur parent syndrome" (or CPS). It occurs when parents drive their kids to the practices, games, rehearsals, scrimmages, swim and track meets or birthday parties. Parents then sit at those events for hours at a time. This syndrome can flair up anywhere from two to seven days or evenings per week. Time you could spend standing up or walking is spent sitting on a bleacher, on the sidelines or at a dance studio—you get the picture. You're thinking, *is she telling me to kick my kids to the curb?* No. Just don't waste ten to fifteen hours per week sitting while waiting for the kids. Get walking instead!

- **Walk the football and track fields**

Walk during the practices, weather permitting. Walk around the school. If the hallways are not closed to the public, walk the halls during your kids' basketball or gymnastics practices. Swim and track meets? We all know how long those meets last and how much time passes in between each event. So, again, get busy walking around the school and parking lot. Usually, there's at least one more field at the school. Use it!

- **Invite other parents to walk with you**

Bring others along. Learn to walk and talk. If they do not join you, do not concern yourself, I repeat, do not concern yourself with what other parents think. Handle your business. Get those steps in. Get busy getting slender, healthy, and cute again! Now some of you have just enough time to drop one kid off before having to pick up another one, and so on, and squeezing in steps during those chauffeur hours is not realistic. Revisit your hourly schedule to ensure that you have identified other moments throughout the day that will afford you the time and the opportunity to reach a minimum of ten thousand steps per day. *You have the power to make it happen!*

➢ *Exercise class and the fitness center*

Exercise classes, going to the gym, workout videos, and other routines are great ways to burn calories, build muscle, stimulate fat burning, and improve your cardiovascular condition if you have the time, the money, the discipline, and the commitment to stick with it. If you do, go for it. Be consistent The muscle you build stimulates our metabolism, replaces fat, and helps control insulin levels.

Many of the suggestions in this chapter are for those who have tried the gym, the classes, the Zumba, and the videos and have fallen off of the wagon and regained the weight. Going to Zumba for the rest of your life simply was not realistic. Some of you might still be paying for the gym membership, although you haven't been to the gym in four months. We've all been there. The point is, these structured exercise programs are fine and effective if you stick with them... but they are not the only route to slimville.

OLD WAYS ARE PASSED AWAY!

Below is the old/new list reflecting what we USED to do before now, along with what WE WILL ACCOMPLISH from this day forward!

<u>Old</u>	<u>New</u>
Sitting all day	Standing up every twenty to thirty minutes to walk or do deskercises for at least two minutes
Doing one workout per day	Taking two to three fifteen minute walks (even if just at home) along with your workout
Being embarrassed by your size	Remembering that you are fearfully and wonderfully made... and that the weight now has an expiration date!
Not moving because of knee or back pain	Wearing a back or knee brace; taping knees with orthopedic tape; icing before/after walk
Having no energy	Drinking a glass of water before your walk and getting enough sleep at night
Having no time for physical activity	Making time!
Not walking because no one will join you	Walking anyway

****

JUSTFORME TIP: I Have Bad Knees and Can't Walk!

Many of you have suffered knee or even back degeneration for one reason or another or because you carry extra weight. I know many individuals who suffer day in and day out, struggling to walk for just five pain-filled minutes, let alone ten thousand steps. If I'm talking to you, one of the most important things you can do is to work toward increasing your mobility as much as possible. This might involve going to the doctor for a referral for physical therapy. The therapist will create an exercise or rehabilitation plan for you. Attend all of your therapy sessions and set aside time to do the exercises. If you are unable to make all of your therapy sessions, explain your circumstance to the therapist and have her write out your plan for the next several weeks or even months. Additionally, ask the therapist for upper-body exercises along with the exercises provided to restore your leg or knee strength and mobility.

****

CHAPTER 11

The Seven Diet-Deadly (Tox) Sins

Do you not know that you are GOD's temple?
1 Corinthians 3:16

P ut on your mask and protective gear...

We know by now that studies point to a possible link between obesogens and obesity. "Some scientists have coined this term for chemicals that may promote obesity, which increase the number of fat cells and slow our metabolism."[xxxii] Obesogens are found not just in our foods. *They are found in personal-care products, and they include phthalates, sodium lauryl sulfates, parabens and other substances added to our shampoos, conditioners, lotions, and hand creams, among other beauty products.* Obesogens include (but are not limited to) antibiotics, hormones, monosodium glutamate, and even stress. The more we lessen the toxic load, the easier it will be to lose the weight and keep it off. Here are the *JustForMeDiet's* seven diet deadly (tox)sins:

1. BPA (and Other Bisphenols)

The much-debated bisphenol A (BPA) is a chemical found in plastic water bottles, scores of can linings, milk carton linings, plastics, and in many brands of microwavable food packaging, among other places. While the debate rages on as to whether BPA causes cancer, many researchers agree that BPA is an endocrine disruptor that has been linked to obesity, diabetes, fibroid tumors, breast cancer, and a decrease in testosterone in boys. Until the debate is resolved, I prefer to work at decreasing the amount of BPA and other bisphenols in my life. Citing multiple studies, the nutritionists at Authority Nutrition observed that: "*BPA is structured in a way that mimics the natural hormone estradiol, a female sex hormone...BPA increased both the number of fat cells, as well as the amount of fat that the fat cells produced and held on to... BPA exposure has also been linked to insulin resistance, cardiovascular disease, diabetes, neurological disorders, thyroid dysfunction, cancer, genital malformations and a lot more.*"[xxxiii]

These days, I use BPA-free water containers. Every morning I fill a forty-ounce stainless-steel water bottle from the refrigerator's purified water dispenser to take with me to work. I make every effort to purchase products that come in glass. Peanut butter in plastic or glass? I'll choose the glass. Salad dressing in glass or plastic? Glass, thank you. Cans with BPA-lining or BPA-free labeled cans? Yes, I pay the extra dollar for the BPA-free label. According to www.wordpress.com, cans from these companies are BPA-free: Amy's, Bionaturae, Eden Foods, Fresh & Easy, Native Forest, Nijiya Market, Muir Glen, and Trader Joe's. I am sure there are others out there.

Will this changeover happen overnight? Of course not. We can try, however, to limit our exposure by purchasing more items packaged in glass, drinking more water out of glass, filtering tap water, and cooking our meals on the stove and in the oven instead of nuking (did I say nuking? I meant microwaving) our food in plastic or Styrofoam containers. Alternatively, when microwaving is unavoidable, we can cook our food in glass or paper dishes.

2.   **Endocrine-Disrupting Chemicals in Toiletries.**

Parabens, phthalates, and sodium lauryl sulfates are just a few examples of chemicals found in many of our soaps, shampoos, conditioners, products used by our hair stylists, perfumes, colognes, and lotions. The chemicals fall into the obesogen category because they are thought to be endocrine disruptors that adversely affect weight. I know it is not easy to part with products you've been using for a lifetime and to seek out and try new products. Over time, however, you'll be able to transition to less-toxic products. The more we buy the nontoxic brands, the more the manufacturers will get the message—*when you eliminate the toxic chemicals from these products, we'll start buying them again.*

3. Pesticides, Fungicides, and Herbicides

Remember the landmark study published in the British Journal of Nutrition that revealed a higher antioxidant content in organic produce than in the non-organic produce? That 18-69 percent differential was huge for me. This means that unless your fruits or veggies are organic, you might be receiving a significantly reduced level of the antioxidants needed to fight disease and inflammation and boost your metabolism. My question is, why pay the extra money and not reap the benefits? Remember, less inflammation means less belly fat and disease.

According to www.sourcewatch.org, the Environmental Working Group's "Dirty Dozen" foods that typically have high-pesticide residues (and probably should be eaten organically if possible) include *apples, celery, strawberries, peaches, spinach, imported nectarines, imported grapes, raspberries, potatoes, bell peppers, domestic blueberries, lettuce, kale, and collard greens.* Because I increased my intake of these foods over the past couple of years, I wanted to make sure I wasn't hurting myself in the process by increasing the toxic load brought by the pesticides, fungicides, and herbicides that accompanied this increase. On the other hand, the following foods are on the lower end of the toxic spectrum: *onions, pineapple, avocado, asparagus, frozen sweet peas, mangos, cantaloupe (domestic), grapefruit, cabbage, sweet potatoes, and mushrooms.*

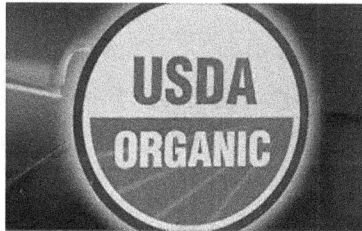

Many of these foods have peels or skins that protect the interior edible portion. For produce with no protective peel, pesticide, herbicide and fungicide residue is often found on the produce or in the soil that nourishes the produce. Or, the substances are genetically engineered into the DNA of the plant.[xxxiv] Most of the produce and food products I buy are **USDA-Certified Organic** or **NON-GMO Project Verified.** Although, ounce for ounce, organic produce often costs more than the non-organic produce, I have learned to cut expenses in other areas (can you say, "staycation?") to free up funds to spend on organic food.

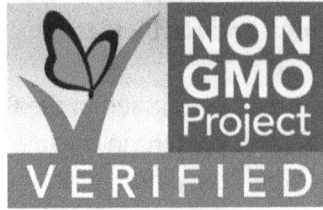

*Examples of GMO foods: soy, corn, cottonseed oils
and products, sugar, and white potatoes*

The USDA estimated that, in 2012, over 90 percent of all soy, 85 percent of the corn, over 90 percent of the cotton (cottonseed oil is used in many mayonnaises, salad dressings, and marinades), and around 95 percent of the sugar beets grown in the United States were genetically engineered. Sugar beets account for 50 percent of the white sugar sold in this country. We have been eating GMOs in increasing amounts for nearly twenty years. If your diet consists of a lot of corn, soy, potato, sugar, or packaged foods, or you eat out frequently, you probably are eating a great deal of GMOs. What does this mean for the *JustForMeDiet*? Again, according to recent studies, pesticides, herbicides, and fungicides—whether sprayed or genetically engineered into the DNA of the plant—are believed to lead to a reduction in the produce's antioxidant content. Yet, the more antioxidants you eat, the lower your inflammation levels. The lower your inflammation levels, the better chance you have of fighting disease and losing weight.

****

JUSTFORME TIP: I Simply Can't Afford Organic Food!

As one who buys organic food as often as possible, I understand the concern. At the same time, we are quick to say we cannot afford organic produce, but then we spend a chunk of change on fast food, pizza, processed snacks, and quick, microwavable, plastic-wrapped meals. Below I compare the cost of the typical fast-food dinner to the cost of a dinner made from organic groceries:

COST OF FAST-FOOD DINNER for a family of four:
Two big burgers or chicken sandwiches, small cheeseburger,
six chicken nuggets, two medium and two small fries, and two
medium and two small sodas:
TOTAL: $28.00

COST OF ORGANIC FOOD DINNER for a family of four:
A four-pound organic chicken @ $2.49/lb. at the discount bulk store ($10.00),
organic brown rice (bag lasts two to three meals) ($3.50),
one pound organic broccoli ($2.50), and one-half gallon
organic milk ($4.00)
TOTAL: $20.00
****

In the example above, not only do you save eight dollars, but there might be leftover chicken for lunch. The milk will last for a couple of days, and the bag of brown rice will net you one or two more meals. Moreover, the organic chicken contained no antibiotics or hormones, nor was it fed genetically modified food. The rice contained no trans fat, and the broccoli was USDA certified organic, meaning the antioxidant level was likely higher.

WINNER: ORGANIC FOOD!

4. Monosodium Glutamate

First and foremost, monosodium glutamate (MSG) is found not just in Chinese food. It is used to flavor chips, seafood seasonings, meat tenderizers, broths, and many other food products. You should conduct your online research to determine what foods contain MSG. In the meantime, you should know that an NIH report links MSG to an increase in glucose and insulin.[xxxv] It gets worse:

> It has been shown, that MSG (120 mg/kg/day), in combination with aspartame, elevated body weight and caused [a]2.3-fold increase in fasting blood glucose compared to standard chow and also caused increased insulin resistance during the Insulin Tolerance Test compared to aspartame.[xxxvi]

So, those MSG-laden chips together with that diet cola are quite the dynamic duo! As such, MSG lands a spot on the seven diet deadly (tox)sins list.

5. Artificial Growth Hormones

We've all gone to the grocery store and have seen the labels on the milk or meat that say, "No rBGH" or "Grass Fed." rBGH refers to growth hormones given to cows. And that "No rBGH" label is usually accompanied by another label that induces sticker shock—the price! Do I want to pay substantially more for milk, yogurt, or meat from grass-fed cows? Well, it appears that rBGH increases insulin in the body, and the debate persists over its link to breast and other cancers. Organic cow and almond milk, particularly the brands with vitamin D and calcium added, are my preferred substitutes for cow's milk treated with rBGH. One last thought: grass fed is a good thing, but that label alone doesn't tell me if the grass has been sprayed with pesticides or herbicides. USDA-Certified Organic clears up the confusion for me.

6. Antibiotics Given to Animals We Eat

As is commonly known, antibiotics are routinely added to grain feed to fatten up (uh, I mean, "stimulate" the growth of) livestock in America. This practice has led to the rise of antibiotic-resistant bacteria. According to the CDC, "*Resistant bacteria in food-producing animals are of particular concern. Food animals serve as a reservoir of resistant pathogens and resistance mechanisms that can directly, or indirectly, result in antibiotic resistant infections in humans. For example, resistant bacteria may be transmitted to humans through the foods we eat.*" ("Antibiotic Use in Food-Producing Animals," National Antimicrobial Resistance Monitoring System, September, 2014.) We are eating resistant bacteria from the meat and dairy derived from animals given antibiotics. Seriously, you can't make this stuff up!

Antibiotics, as we also know, destroy good gut bacteria along with the bad bacteria it is intended for, thus compromising our immune system. This is why our doctors tell us to eat yogurt when they prescribe a course of antibiotics because the yogurt, as the doctors explain, contains probiotics that help restore the good bacteria that we really do need for a strong immune system. The problem occurs when you regularly eat meat, yogurt, and cheese, and drink milk from cows that are given antibiotics. Is that like taking penicillin every day of your life? I don't know.

As if that wasn't bad enough, recent studies (feel free to do your own research) link the gut bacteria imbalance caused by the antibiotics—including that which passes directly from the animals to us—to diabetes and obesity. (Read "The Fat Drug," *The New York Times*, March 8, 2014; and "Livestock Antibiotics Could Have Contributed to Human Obesity" Nick Collins, UK's *The Telegraph*, August 22, 2012). Let's review the lesson:

Cow + antibiotics = FAT COW! Man + FAT COW = FAT MAN!

Adds up to me!

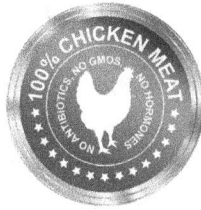

Why we prefer organic chicken (and their eggs!)
Poultry is another category of animals that are given antibiotics and hormones. Again, in the grocery store, we see "free range" or "cage free" on the chicken packages and egg cartons. If you are not from the farm, you might not know what that really means. Okay, I'll just speak for myself. I had no clue! So I investigated. The idea is that free-range chickens are free to roam and eat what chickens eat naturally, such as bugs, worms, grass, vegetables, and flowers, as opposed to food consisting of nonorganic grain. Free range or cage free means that the chickens are not raised in a cage and instead can roam about, but there's no indication of any vegetation for them to eat. Most studies compare the nutritional values of organic and other eggs and conclude that the organic eggs contain more nutrients and less cholesterol and saturated fat. At the end of the day, you want more health bang for your buck.

****

JUSTFORME TIP: How Do I Know Which Foods Contain GMOs?
You know by selecting USDA-Certified Organic or NON-GMO Certified foods. When I see "corn, soy, sugar, canola, or white potatoes" in the ingredient list, unless I see "organic" or "GMO-free," I assume that the food contains GMOs.

****

7. **Stress!**

> **And now, dear brothers and sisters, one final thing.**
> **Fix your thoughts on what is true, and honorable, and right,**
> **and pure, and lovely, and admirable. Think about things that are excellent**
> **and worthy of praise.**
> **Philippians 4:8 (NLT)**

Stress makes the "diet deadly (tox)sin list" because of the impact it has on our weight and life expectancy. Who isn't facing some measure of stress, whether in the home, on the job, in our finances, with our health, and our families? We all feel stressed to some degree. Stress actually leads to a release of cortisol, the fight or flight hormone in our bloodstream. That's a good thing if you're being chased in a horror movie. But if it is released on a daily basis, it leads to an imbalance in our hormones and a glucose increase in our bloodstream, leading to fat buildup in the belly, among other conditions.

I do not know what your stressors are, but I do know that they can feel overwhelming at times. Worrying, however, will not fix the problem. Instead, worry only adds to stress, and stress adds pounds to the body and subtracts years from your life. Stress is at the root of much inflammation in the body, which leads to belly fat. It turns out that the Apostle Paul offered spiritual *and* medical advice when he instructed us to think on things that are of lovely and admirable. Instead of worrying, I suggest that you pray about the things that stress you, seek counseling if necessary, laugh (good medicine!) as often as possible, and walk more to relieve stress. It also helps to get enough sleep at night. Above all, put your trust in the Lord and know that all things are working together for your good.

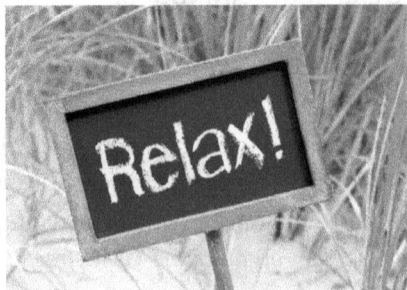

Finally, we all fall prey to stress eating. Remember: sugar, fast foods, and fried foods are inflammatory—inflammation triggers more stress and stress triggers more inflammation, perpetuating an endless cycle. No worries—If you are stressed, relax. Know that GOD is in control. Take five minutes and remember the last time GOD delivered you. Instead of reaching for the cookies (they should no longer be in your cabinet, by the way), have some guacamole. Or, since your cupboard, car, and purse are stocked with healthy bars, reach for one of them to calm the stressed-out savage beast. Drink a glass of water—it just might do the trick. A cup of chamomile tea is a great stress reliever at bedtime (but don't drink it and drive!)

CHAPTER 12

Reaching the Finish Line...Permanently!

But one thing I do, forgetting what is behind, I press toward the goal...
PHILIPPIANS 3:13–14

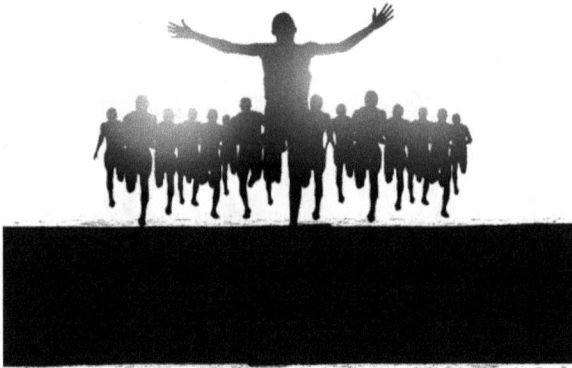

PLATEAUS

Needless to say (but I'll tell you anyway), I hit a plateau a few times during my weight-loss odyssey. It seems like the first thirty pounds just melted off. They actually did. Then the weight loss slowed to a halt for a little while. I began to understand my body a bit more and how it worked. It needed to adjust to the new me and find a new rhythm. After about three weeks, the next four to five pounds fell off, and then my body rested again. A month later, the next four to five pounds fell off. And so on.

After losing the first thirty-five pounds, it seemed as if I wasn't going to lose any more weight. To be clear, I was within the "normal" BMI range, but I was at the higher end of the range and I wanted to be in the middle range. The last ten pounds, I discovered, are the toughest ten of them all. Nonetheless, they became my past. Below I show you how.

LOSING THE LAST TEN

Although these tenacious ten hold on like a pit bull, there's no need to worry. You can, and will, rid yourself of these extra pounds. It just takes making a few more adjustments, such as taking your movement to the next level and jump-starting your metabolism by cutting back on some starchy carbs for a brief while. Below are the last ten steps that dissolved my *last ten pounds*. Maybe they'll work for you, too!

- **Choose the right time frame**. Don't plan on losing the last ten pounds during your seven-day anniversary cruise. Be realistic. There are several occasions during the year, such as when you're on vacation or celebrating anniversaries, birthdays, Thanksgiving, and Christmas, when weight loss is tough. For me, the goal simply is not to gain, or not to gain more than two pounds and then offload them when the season or event passes.
- **Get buy-in from your family**. We've already discussed how our family's food shopping, cooking, and eating habits can sometimes hinder us. As long as the food is in the house and staring at you from the top of the fridge, you probably will eat it (I'll speak for myself). Not only must you readjust your *own* shopping habits but you must readjust the shopping habits of everyone in the household; otherwise, your efforts are sabotaged. For example, I might escape the grocery store with no cookies in my bags, but if my family members later come home with those cookies, I'm a goner. I repeat, I'm a goner. Therefore, sit down with the offenders and get their buy-in. From my own experience, blame won't get you very far. Trust me, it's better to praise them by telling them how wonderful they are and how you simply can't do it without their invaluable assistance. Use enough sugar in your speech to trigger diabetic shock. This next suggestion is controversial—ask them to remove the temptation from the house and keep it in their cars or otherwise hidden from you. If they don't cooperate, toss the cookies into the garbage can. Point made.

- **Return to ground zero**. This suggestion involves dusting off the meal plans from the early days that jump-started your weight-loss success. My weight loss started off fast and furiously. I lost eleven pounds in the first month. I drank two to three smoothies per week, ate oatmeal three or four mornings per week, ate no bread or bread products, no rice, pasta, or white potatoes, no juices, and no fried foods hardly at all during the first couple of months. By the time I was ready to lose the last ten, complacency had set in. I had stopped adding up how many carbohydrate, protein, or even "healthy" fat grams I was eating. I would reach for some guacamole and chips and go to town. When I was done, the organic tortilla chip bag and the four-serving guacamole bowl were gone. Yes, I learned you can binge on healthy food. Lesson learned! For the last lap, to paraphrase, I needed to return to the "cross where I first saw the light and the burden of my *weight* rolled away."

- **Eliminate the creeps**. The what? Yes, eliminate the old ways that have crept back into your diet and lifestyle. This involves taking a fresh look at what you have been eating and where the dietary and lifestyle complacency have set in. At the forty-pound-loss-point plateau, I needed to take a fresh look at what my daily eating, walking, and movement habits had been over the past several weeks. My "creeps" were: (1) lower water intake. My usual eight to ten glasses of water or herbal tea had crept downward to five to six glasses; (2) increased bread intake; (3) fewer steps taken since I eliminated evening walks because of the *darkness and cold that had descended upon the land* (daylight savings time and winter); and (4) increased sitting time at a computer without rising.

- **Fast**. Once per week, usually on Sunday after a 3:00 p.m. dinner, I fasted for eighteen hours. I did not eat again until 9:00 a.m. on Monday. This short fast gave my digestive system a break and allowed my body to dispose of some fat and the extra glucose that was racing around in my blood. I found that I thought more clearly, slept better, and was truly refreshed the next day. Fasting is a surefire scale mover!

- **Add one more short walk.** If you walk every day for thirty minutes, and are standing up every thirty minutes or so to walk for two minutes, try adding one more thirty-minute walk three to four times per week. Also, if you have a treadmill, start using it to assist with burning the last ten pounds. I walked at lunch during the day, and I walked on the treadmill twice per week for about fifteen to twenty minutes.

- **Take additional steps**. If you consistently have been walking your ten thousand steps per day, it might be time to bump up that number to twelve to fifteen thousand steps for three additional days per week. My scale began to move downward again when I increased the steps to fifteen thousand for a few extra days per week.

- **Consider a meal replacement smoothie once or twice per week.** This works really well on Saturday or Sunday, when you have the time to make it with the right ingredients. *Make your own!* If I'm replacing a meal with my smoothie, I usually add the following ingredients to the blender: a half-scoop of organic undenatured whey protein, seven to eight walnuts, a half-cup of berries, and one cup of greens/broccoli. I might add some pineapple mint and cilantro from the garden. Sometimes I add half a cup of low-fat organic Greek yogurt, along with coconut water. If I add the yogurt, I do not use protein powder. I also avoid adding fruit juices, with one or two exceptions. I might add one ounce of tart cherry juice because it tastes so good and is loaded with melatonin, a very powerful antioxidant. I occasionally add no more than two ounces of low-sugar orange juice. More often than not, I add berries, mangos, bananas, and apples instead of juice. As you can see, I throw the kitchen sink into my smoothies, and no two smoothies are alike. I'm just not that consistent, sorry. That's someone else's diet book!

- **Add soups and teas to your diet**. I'm not talking about store-bought soup. These are soups you make at home on a Saturday or Sunday afternoon, which last three to four days. I'm talking about the soup you make with a whole cut-up organic chicken, some celery, onions, carrots, and other veggies, as well as, garlic, cilantro, turmeric, rosemary, parsley, basil, a tad bit of salt, black and crushed red peppers, along with other herbs and spices. In addition to the soups, some teas, including green tea, help boost the metabolism—the body's fat-burning process. I find that when I drink herbal teas throughout the day, I'm simply not that hungry. During the spring and summer, make iced tea with flavored herbal teas, but do not add sugar. Over time, your taste buds will learn to enjoy the flavor of the unsweetened herbal tea.

- **Increase deskercises and "housercises."** To help drop the last couple of pounds, I incorporated a few more "deskercises" while at work and "housercises"(sounds better than "housework") while at home. Those included walking up and down the stairs, hand scrubbing the floors, and washing walls and cars. Remember "wax on-wax off"? Bouncing on the mini trampoline a few more times during the evening will help. You can even use soup cans to help build arm muscles.

****

JUSTFORME TIP: *I Can't Fast Because I Take Medication with Food.*
Ask your physician whether you can fast, even if only in between meals. The eighteen-hour fast can be accomplished easily during the hours between dinner and breakfast the next morning. If you must "break" it for medical purposes, by all means do so. Always check with your doctor if you are on medication before fasting for any length of time.

****

KEEPING IT OFF

People have asked me how I have managed to keep the weight off. The truth is, fear is a great motivator for me. Now that I have seen with my own eyes what diabetes, cancer, and obesity have done to the people around me, I have been scared straight! Is it too late to reverse the damage that five million French fries, four million slices of bread, three million cookies, two million glasses of orange juice, strawberry lemonade refills, and one million slices of pizza have done to our bodies? I don't think so. Without a doubt, we certainly can slow the decline and start the healing process today!

The road to keeping it off begins with truly understanding that this journey isn't so much about weight loss or being able to fit into those jeans. It is about making a lifestyle change to improve your quality of life and to prevent life-threatening diseases. The foods and food additives we've subsisted on during the past two to three decades have been slowly poisoning us. The weight is just a by-product of the internal toxicity. The link between the toxic additives, preservatives, and chemicals found in many foods currently sold at the grocery store, and obesity, diabetes, and cancer makes it easier to pay the few extra dollars for the organic brands or to just say no when the pizza is passed around. Do I get it right 100 percent of the time? Of course not (remember those cookies), but my choices are improving daily. I like the new me—the one with:

- ✓ Three times the energy I had when I was carrying around an extra forty-five pounds
- ✓ Fewer senior moments (*come on, now—you didn't think they all were gone, did you?*)
- ✓ Far fewer knee or back aches
- ✓ A stronger immune system...Oh, and I almost forgot—
- ✓ A slimmer, trimmer body!

So, keeping the weight off involves the following FAB FIVE tips:

- **Stay vigilant about your food choices**. Now that you have created your *JustForMeDiet* grocery list and shopping guides, stay on track with your food purchases. When you shop, purchase a full week's worth of *JustForMeDiet* snacks to have with you at all times because there will be unhealthy alternatives everywhere you go, every single day. Similar to the measures taken by those battling alcohol or other addictions, this needs to be a lifetime state of vigilance. Just as you wouldn't ever leave the back door of your home unlocked at night (unless you live on a deserted island), don't leave the door to your health unguarded. Again, when holidays come around, when family members come to town or when you must travel for work, exercise your due diligence and prepare in advance.
- **Weigh yourself once per week**. This is called nipping the weight gain in the bud (or is it butt?). Again, by weighing yourself, you catch the creeping weight gain before it gets out of hand.
- **Make adjustments when necessary**. If you notice an uptick in pounds after the weekly weigh in, you might want to adjust a few things. Consult the "losing the last ten" section and implement the suggestions.
- **Plan ahead for special occasions and holidays**. This step involves looking at your calendar to mark upcoming food events. They come around every year. Plan to eat as healthfully as possible during the pre- and post days. Make sure your pantry is stocked with the bodyguards. In fact, put them on the counter so you reach for them before leaving home for the high-sugar, high-carb event. Fit in a few thousand additional steps on the day of the event.
- **Share your diet with family and friends**. You've heard the saying, "Each one, teach one." Well, I say "Each one, teach one or two—or seven or ten!" As long as all of your friends and family members eat fattening and unhealthy foods, regularly eat out, or constantly prepare

diet-destroying meals, you will face a relentless onslaught of daily and nightly temptation. Moreover, everyone around you will insist that you have lost enough weight, that you are "wasting away," and that it is okay to reward yourself or cheat a little. Remember: You know what your goal is. It cannot be set by anyone but you and your physician. Friends asked me, "What's the point, if you can't enjoy yourself?" Or how about, "You need something bad to eat every now and then for balance." Trust me: ignoring or politely [or not] responding to the remarks was difficult for a while.

On the other hand, if you bring your loved ones along with you on this journey, not only will you ease the pressure and temptation that eventually will set you back, but you also will help them make healthier choices to improve their lives. I cannot enjoy my improved health if everyone around me is still suffering. By helping your loved ones lose the weight, you help them defeat obesity, lower their heart disease, diabetes, and cancer risks, and ultimately reach a state of wholeness. That's love.

CONCLUSION

Congratulations! You now have the tools to create your own *JustForMeDiet* plan. As I am sure you have realized, this book really is about shedding our old ways of doing things – whether our inactivity or our refined food diet – and adopting a healthier lifestyle. This healthier you must include the spiritual, mental and emotional you. Will you fall off the wagon occasionally? Of course you will. No worries. When you do fall, get back up by remembering your bodyguards. Make adjustments the next day. Add a few thousand steps to compensate for the damage done. Never be afraid to ask for help, starting with asking GOD to strengthen you, help you to exercise self-control, and to remove temptation from your path. We are all in this boat together so bring others along. Let's gently encourage each other. None of us has all of the answers, so let's compare notes and share best practices.

I encourage you to be an active participant, not just with your weight loss, but with your health in general. Access and read the reports and studies referenced in the endnotes. They are worth reading and will broaden your understanding of your health challenges *and* solutions—they certainly broadened my "health horizon."

I close with this: it is time to get busy losing weight, being healthier, feeling better, regaining high-octane energy levels, and, with GOD's help, transforming yourself into the fearfully and wonderfully made person He created—someone who is *prospering in all things, in health, just as your soul prospers* (3 John 2 NKJV).

It can be done!

NOTES

i   "About BMI for Adults." Centers for Disease Control and Prevention. February 23, 2015. Accessed March 9, 2015. http://www.cdc.gov/healthy-weight/assessing/bmi/adult_bmi/index.html.

ii   "Fitness and Nutrition." Womenshealth.gov. June 17, 2008. Accessed March 9, 2015. http://www.womenshealth.gov/fitness-nutrition/nutri-tion-basics/carbohydrates.html.

iii   "Sleep and Chronic Disease." Centers for Disease Control and Prevention. July 1, 2013. Accessed March 9, 2015. http://www.cdc.gov/sleep/about_sleep/chronic_disease.htm.

iv   Blosser, Fred. "Body Clock Disruption, Linked With Travel Across Time Zones, Seen in Study of Flight Attendants." Centers for Disease Control and Prevention. August 6, 2012. Accessed March 10, 2015. http://www.cdc.gov/niosh/updates/bodyclok.html.

v   "Physical Activity for a Healthy Weight." Centers for Disease Control and Prevention. September 13, 2011. Accessed March 10, 2015. http://www.cdc.gov/healthyweight/physical_activity/index.html?s_cid=govD_dnpao_006.; "EPublications." Physical Activity (exercise) Fact Sheet. February 26, 2009. Accessed March 10, 2015. http://womenshealth.gov/publications/our-publications/fact-sheet/physical-activity.html.

vi   Your physician or nutritionist is a required partner in determining how many proteins, carbs, fats, sugars and fiber grams you should be consuming. When you have your pre-*JustForMeDiet* medical exam, ask your physician to determine your personal macronutrient ranges.

vii   Age, activity level, and even muscle mass, among other things, are variables that can increase or decrease your protein needs.

viii   "Dietary Reference Intakes for Energy, Carbohydrate, Fiber, Fat, Fatty Acids, Cholesterol, Protein, and Amino Acids - Institute of Medicine." Dietary

Reference Intakes. September 5, 2002. Accessed March 11, 2015. http://www.iom.edu/Reports/2002/Dietary-Reference-Intakes-for-Energy-Carbohydrate-Fiber-Fat-Fatty-Acids-Cholesterol-Protein-and-Amino-Acids.aspx.

ix   "Basics About Diabetes." Centers for Disease Control and Prevention. October 21, 2014. Accessed March 10, 2015. http://www.cdc.gov/diabetes/basics/diabetes.html.

x   "National Diabetes Information Clearinghouse (NDIC)." Insulin Resistance and Prediabetes. September 10, 2014. Accessed March 10, 2015. http://diabetes.niddk.nih.gov/dm/pubs/insulinresistance/.

xi   Gunnars, Kris. "A Simple Way to Fix The Hormones That Make You Fat." Authority Nutrition. January 12, 2014. Accessed March 10, 2015. http://authoritynutrition.com/fix-the-hormones-that-make-you-fat/.

xii   Song, YJ, M. Sawamura, K. Ikeda, S. Igawa, and Y. Yamori. "Soluble Dietary Fibre Improves Insulin Sensitivity by Increasing Muscle GLUT-4 Content in Stroke-prone Spontaneously Hypertensive Rats." National Center for Biotechnology Information. January 1, 2000. Accessed March 10, 2015. http://www.ncbi.nlm.nih.gov/pubmed/10696527

xiii   Gunnars, Kris. "9 Ways That Processed Foods Are Slowly Killing People." Authority Nutrition. January 15, 2014. Accessed March 10, 2015. http://authoritynutrition.com/9-ways-that-processed-foods-are-killing-people/.

xiv   Gunnars, Kris. "Daily Intake of Sugar - How Much Sugar Should You Eat Per Day?" Authority Nutrition. April 24, 2013. Accessed March 10, 2015. http://authoritynutrition.com/how-much-sugar-per-day.

xv   MSG and all its aliases, you know, natural flavors, spices, soy protein isolate, etc. are considered neurotoxins (look it up!)—stuff we should not be eating and definitely *do not want to give our children*!

xvi   Macronutrients include carbohydrates, fiber, fat, fatty acids, cholesterol, protein, and amino acids.

xvii   "Protein." Centers for Disease Control and Prevention. October 4, 2012. Accessed March 10, 2015. http://www.cdc.gov/nutrition/everyone/basics/protein.html#sthash.wHwVlfEP.dpuf.

xviii   "Soluble vs. Insoluble Fiber: MedlinePlus Medical Encyclopedia." Medline Plus. September 2, 2012. Accessed March 10, 2015. http://www.nlm.nih.gov/medlineplus/ency/article/002136.htm.

xix   Ibid.

xx   "High-Fiber Food Guide - Meta Wellness." Fiberlicious Food Guide. January 1, 2012. Accessed March 10, 2015. http://www.metawellness.com/en-us/articles/fiber/fiberlicious-food-guide.

xxi   "Polyunsaturated fats and Monounsaturated fats" Centers for Disease Control and Prevention. September 27, 2012. Accessed March 10, 2015. http://www.cdc.gov/nutrition/everyone/basics/fat/unsaturatedfat.html

xxii   Keep in mind that some fish, such as tuna and swordfish, have more mercury than others, so I limit tuna and high-mercury fish meals to once or twice per month.

xxiii   "Wild caught" means it was not farm raised or fed genetically modified soy or corn products.

xxiv   "Trans Fat." Centers for Disease Control and Prevention. January 8, 2014. Accessed March 10, 2015. http://www.cdc.gov/nutrition/everyone/basics/fat/transfat.html.

xxv   Higdon, Jane, and Victoria Drake. "Isothiocyanates." Linus Pauling Institute at Oregon State University. September 1, 2005. Accessed March 10, 2015. http://lpi.oregonstate.edu/infocenter/phytochemicals/isothio/#glucosinolates.

xxvi   Barański, Marcin, Dominika Średnicka-Tober, Nikolaos Volakakis, Chris Seal, Roy Sanderson, Gavin Stewart, Charles Benbrook, Bruno Biavati, Emilia Markellou, Charilaos Giotis, Joanna Gromadzka-Ostrowska, Ewa

Rembiałkowska, Krystyna Skwarło-Sońta, Raija Tahvonen, Dagmar Janovská, Urs Niggli, Philippe Nicot, and Carlo Leifert. "Higher Antioxidant and Lower Cadmium Concentrations and Lower Incidence of Pesticide Residues in Organically Grown Crops: A Systematic Literature Review and Meta-analyses." *British Journal of Nutrition* 112, no. 5 (2014): 794-811.

xxvii   "What Counts as a Cup?" Centers for Disease Control and Prevention. June 18, 2012. Accessed March 10, 2015. http://www.cdc.gov/nutrition/everyone/fruitsvegetables/cup.html.

xxviii   Cho, Jae - Hyoung. "Balsamic Vinegar Improves High Fat-Induced Beta Cell Dysfunction via Beta Cell ABCA1." *Diabetes and Metabolism Journal* 36, no. 36(5) (2012): 388–389.

Gunnars, Kris. "Why Is Fiber Good For You? The Crunchy Truth." Authority Nutrition. November 28, 2013. Accessed March 10, 2015. http://authoritynutrition.com/why-is-fiber-good-for-you/.

Gunnars, Kris. "6 Proven Benefits of Apple Cider Vinegar (No. 3 Is Best)." Authority Nutrition. June 22, 2014. Accessed March 10, 2015. http://authoritynutrition.com/6-proven-health-benefits-of-apple-cider-vinegar.

Gunnars, Kris. "10 Proven Benefits of Green Tea (No. 3 Is Very Impressive)." Authority Nutrition. September 2, 2013. Accessed March 10, 2015. http://authoritynutrition.com/top-10-evidence-based-health-benefits-of-green-tea/.

xxix   "Water: Meeting Your Daily Fluid Needs." Centers for Disease Control and Prevention. October 10, 2012. Accessed March 10, 2015. http://www.cdc.gov/nutrition/everyone/basics/water.html.

xxx   Gunnars, Kris. "How Much Water Should You Drink Per Day?" Authority Nutrition. October 24, 2013. Accessed March 10, 2015. http://authoritynutrition.com/how-much-water-should-you-drink-per-day/.

xxxi   Pronk, Nicolaas, Abigail Katz, Marcia Lowry, and Jane Payfer. "Reducing Occupational Sitting Time and Improving Worker Health: The Take-a-Stand Project, 2011." *Preventing Chronic Disease* 9, no. 9:110323 (2012).

xxxii   "SOLVING THE PROBLEM OF CHILDHOOD OBESITY WITHIN A GENERATION." *White House Task Force on Childhood Obesity Report to the President,* 2010.

xxxiii   Gunnars, Kris. "5 Artificial Chemicals That Are Making You Fat (Found in Your Home)." Authority Nutrition. August 5, 2013. Accessed March 10, 2015. http://authoritynutrition.com/5-chemicals-that-are-making-you-fat/.

xxxiv   "Glyphosate." - SourceWatch. September 21, 2012. Accessed March 10, 2015. http://www.sourcewatch.org/index.php/Glyphosate.

xxxv   "MONOSODIUM GLUTAMATE." - National Library of Medicine HSDB Database. October 11, 2007. Accessed March 10, 2015. http://toxnet.nlm.nih.gov/cgi-bin/sis/search/a?dbs hsdb:@term @DOCNO 580).

xxxvi   Husarova, Veronika, and Daniela Ostatnikova. "Monosodium Glutamate Toxic Effects and Their Implications for Human Intake: A Review." *JMED Research* 2013 (2013): 1-12.

APPENDIX A

Body Mass Index Table

Body Mass Index Table 1 of 2

BMI	Normal						Overweight					Obese					
	19	20	21	22	23	24	25	26	27	28	29	30	31	32	33	34	35
Height (inches)	Body Weight (pounds)																
58	91	96	100	105	110	115	119	124	129	134	138	143	148	153	158	162	167
59	94	99	104	109	114	119	124	128	133	138	143	148	153	158	163	168	173
60	97	102	107	112	118	123	128	133	138	143	148	153	158	163	168	174	179
61	100	106	111	116	122	127	132	137	143	148	153	158	164	169	174	180	185
62	104	109	115	120	126	131	136	142	147	153	158	164	169	175	180	186	191
63	107	113	118	124	130	135	141	146	152	158	163	169	175	180	186	191	197
64	110	116	122	128	134	140	145	151	157	163	169	174	180	186	192	197	204
65	114	120	126	132	138	144	150	156	162	168	174	180	186	192	198	204	210
66	118	124	130	136	142	148	155	161	167	173	179	186	192	198	204	210	216
67	121	127	134	140	146	153	159	166	172	178	185	191	198	204	211	217	223
68	125	131	138	144	151	158	164	171	177	184	190	197	203	210	216	223	230
69	128	135	142	149	155	162	169	176	182	189	196	203	209	216	223	230	236
70	132	139	146	153	160	167	174	181	188	195	202	209	216	222	229	236	243
71	136	143	150	157	165	172	179	186	193	200	208	215	222	229	236	243	250
72	140	147	154	162	169	177	184	191	199	206	213	221	228	235	242	250	258
73	144	151	159	166	174	182	189	197	204	212	219	227	235	242	250	257	265
74	148	155	163	171	179	186	194	202	210	218	225	233	241	249	256	264	272
75	152	160	168	176	184	192	200	208	216	224	232	240	248	256	264	272	279
76	156	164	172	180	189	197	205	213	221	230	238	246	254	263	271	279	287

Body Mass Index Table 2 of 2

BMI	Obese										Extreme Obesity								
	36	37	38	39	40	41	42	43	44	45	46	47	48	49	50	51	52	53	54
Height (inches)	Body Weight (pounds)																		
58	172	177	181	186	191	196	201	205	210	215	220	224	229	234	239	244	248	253	258
59	178	183	188	193	198	203	208	212	217	222	227	232	237	242	247	252	257	262	267
60	184	189	194	199	204	209	215	220	225	230	235	240	245	250	255	261	266	271	276
61	190	195	201	206	211	217	222	227	232	238	243	248	254	259	264	269	275	280	285
62	196	202	207	213	218	224	229	235	240	246	251	256	262	267	273	278	284	289	295
63	203	208	214	220	225	231	237	242	248	254	259	265	270	278	282	287	293	299	304
64	209	215	221	227	232	238	244	250	256	262	267	273	279	285	291	296	302	308	314
65	216	222	228	234	240	246	252	258	264	270	276	282	288	294	300	306	312	318	324
66	223	229	235	241	247	253	260	266	272	278	284	291	297	303	309	315	322	328	334
67	230	236	242	249	255	261	268	274	280	287	293	299	306	312	319	325	331	338	344
68	236	243	249	256	262	269	276	282	289	295	302	308	315	322	328	335	341	348	354
69	243	250	257	263	270	277	284	291	297	304	311	318	324	331	338	345	351	358	365
70	250	257	264	271	278	285	292	299	306	313	320	327	334	341	348	355	362	369	376
71	257	265	272	279	286	293	301	308	315	322	329	338	343	351	358	365	372	379	386
72	265	272	279	287	294	302	309	316	324	331	338	346	353	361	368	375	383	390	397
73	272	280	288	295	302	310	318	325	333	340	348	355	363	371	378	386	393	401	408
74	280	287	295	303	311	319	326	334	342	350	358	365	373	381	389	396	404	412	420
75	287	295	303	311	319	327	335	343	351	359	367	375	383	391	399	407	415	423	431
76	295	304	312	320	328	336	344	353	361	369	377	385	394	402	410	418	426	435	443

Source: Adapted from *Clinical Guidelines on the Identification, Evaluation, and Treatment of Overweight and Obesity in Adults: The Evidence Report,* National Institutes of Health, 1998.

APPENDIX B

Macronutrient and Sugar Content of Food (rounded to the nearest half gram)

FOOD	PROTEIN	FIBER	FAT	SUGAR	CARB
Almonds (1/4 cup)	6	4	15	1	6
Almond milk (unsweetened) (2 oz.)	0	0	0	0	0
Apple (medium)	.5	4	.5	19	25
Avocado (1 cup)	3	10	21	1	12
Banana (1)	1.5	3	.5	14	27
Bionaturae elbow or rigatoni noodles (1 serving)	7	6	1.5	1	35
Black beans (1 cup)	15	15	0	0	40
Blueberries (1 cup)	1	4	.5	15	21
Bread (1 slice dbl. fiber)	5	6	1	1	17
Broccoli (1 cup cooked)	4	6	0	2	12
Brussels sprouts (1 cup cooked)	2	2	0	1	6
Cauliflower (1 cup cooked)	2	2	0	1	6
Cheese, Swiss (1 slice)	8	0	8	.5	1.5
Chia seeds (2 tbsp.)	4.5	10	9	0	12
Chicken breast (1/2), boneless, skinless	27	0	1.5	0	0
Corn, (1/2 cup) whole, kernel	2.5	2.5	1	2.5	20.5
Grapes (1/2 cup)	.5	1	0	13	14.5
Guacamole (½ cup)	2	5.5	17	0	10
Kale (1 cup cooked)	2	3	1	2	7
Kidney beans (1 cup)	15	11	1	1	40
Lamb chop-fat trimmed! (3 oz.)	22	0	12	0	0
Lentils (1/2 cup cooked)	9	8	.5	2	20
Lima beans (1/2 cup cooked)	7.5	6.5	.5	2.5	19.5
Mayonnaise (1 tbsp.)	0	0	11	0	0

APPENDIX B Cont'd

Macronutrient and Sugar Content of Food (rounded to the nearest half gram)

FOOD	PROTEIN	FIBER	FAT	SUGAR	CARB
Milk-low fat (2 oz.)	2	0	2	3	3
Oatmeal (3/4 cup)	7.5	6	4.5	1.5	40
Olive oil, extra virgin (1 tbsp.)	0	0	14	0	0
Olive oil, extra virgin (spray)	0	0	5	0	0
Peanuts (1/2 cup)	19.5	6	36	3	12
Peanut butter (2 tbsp.)	8	3	16	2	6
Quinoa, cooked (1/2 cup)	4	2.5	2	1	19.5
Raspberries (1 cup)	1.5	8	1	5.5	15
Rice, brown (1/2 cup)	2.5	2	1	.5	22
Salad (1 cup)	2	2	0	0	5
Salmon fillet, wild caught (4 oz.)	22	0	8	0	.5
Shrimp (3 oz.)	21	0	1.5	0	0
Spinach (½ cup cooked)	2.5	2	0	.5	3.5
Stevia, organic (1 packet)	0	.8	0	0	0
Sweet potato (1 medium)	2	4	0	7	24
Tortilla chips (10)	1.5	1	6	0	17
Tuna, chunk lite packed in oil, drained (2 oz.)	10	0	4.5	0	.5
Tuna, chunk lite packed in water, drained (2 oz.)	10.5	0	0	0	0
Turkey chili with beans (1 cup)	20	7	4.5	6	30
Turkey sausages (2)	6	0	4.6	0	1.5
Turkey slices, lunch meat (2 oz.)	12	0	0	0	0
Vinaigrette, balsamic (2 tbsp.)	0	0	3	5	5
Walnut halves (14)	4	2	18	1	4
Whiting (4 oz.)	20	0	4	0	0
Yogurt, plain low-fat (8 oz.)	10	0	2	15	15
Yogurt, plain low-fat Greek (6 oz.)	17	0	3	4	6.5

APPENDIX C

Schedule of Daily Activities

Record "s" for sedentary or sitting

	Sun	Mon	Tue	Wed	Thu	Fri	Sat
7-8							
8-9							
9-12							
12-1							
1-6							
6-7							
7-9							
9-11							

Revised schedule with more physical activity
Record "w" for walk or workout or "d" for deskercises

	Sun	Mon	Tue	Wed	Thu	Fri	Sat
7–8							
8–9							
9–12							
12–1							
1–6							
6–7							
7–9							
9–11